my cancer year

A SURVIVORSHIP MEMOIR

for Paula,
Josh and Jesse,
forever

my cancer year

A SURVIVORSHIP MEMOIR

curtis pesmen

TATRA PRESS LLC

Also by Curtis Pesmen

How a Man Ages
What She Wants: A Man's Guide to Women and Their Bodies
Your First Year of Marriage
When a Man Turns Forty
Your Prostate Cancer Survivor's Guide

◎ table of contents

Author's Note: Though not exactly born as a blog, a first-person account of a life-threatening colon cancer case appeared over six months' time, in the pages of a national magazine. The public/private cancer case happened to be mine.

The series appears in Chapter 1; excerpts also reappear, as reruns on occasion through the book, for narrative flow. In addition, names of certain survivors and related details have been changed for privacy reasons.

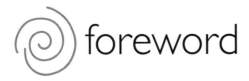 foreword

Sometimes numbers speak louder than words. Sometimes they fairly shout when you don't abbreviate them. So this year, more than 1,600,000 Americans will learn they have cancer. This equates to more than 80 Beyoncé or Bruce Springsteen sold-out shows in New York's Madison Square Garden, in terms of counting bodies. And bodies do count. They're why I wrote this book.

I also wrote it to vent the fears and frustrations of one single cancer patient's life, and to stay connected—to those closest to me, to my friends, to my job, and to the cancer survivor community that I didn't realize I would be part of someday.

As for community, and what it's grown to mean to me, I won't soon forget a letter I received years ago from Sherry Ribble, a health care provider from Honea Path, South Carolina. I didn't know Sherry at all, but she had read some of my words in *Esquire* magazine and said:

> I work at an endoscopy center; we do colonoscopies and
> EGDs, which check the esophagus, stomach and duodenum
> for diseases. It is not unusual for us to do 30 or more cases in
> a day. We see people diagnosed with cancer almost on a daily
> basis. Working as we do, we only see the patients when they
> are diagnosed and their reactions at that moment. Pesmen's

articles have touched me and moved me in so many ways—I
have cried, been angry at the incompetence of his first doctor,
felt guilty because of how little we are able to do for the patient
at that stage, and been amazed at the courage of Pesmen and
his wife to be willing and able to share these intimate moments
with us."

Call me fortunate—and humbled—that I am able to share some
of these personal cancer experiences, still. Here's hoping, then, that
at least a little bit of my "good" cancer year can help you or a loved
one through what surely may become an unforgettable, incredibly
tough, but an also oddly rewarding, time.

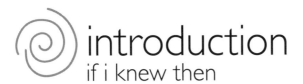

introduction
if i knew then

Of all the scary scenarios and tough talk I heard in the throes of my good cancer year, the most frightening words were not, "You have cancer." No, not those three. The scariest words I heard rolled out of the mouth of a 20-something cancer doc, an apprentice radiation oncology resident who wore a starched white coat while doing Saturday rounds in the sub-floor unit of a busy San Francisco cancer center; who approached my nervous wife, Paula, and me, with a chart in his hands and not a worry line on his forehead and nonchalantly said: "Sorry about the bad news."

Whoa-what? Huh? Epochal. Life-altering (again). Terrifying (anew). Because what he was saying was now worse than what I'd heard six weeks before, which was bad-shock-enough. But back then, when I got my Stage 3, it was delivered by a team of doctors, one of whom had spent more than an hour with us, uninterrupted and early on, laying out what we would face in the weeks and months to come. Back then I'd gotten the news from a team that had compared notes and delivered a diagnosis when we all thought my cancer was, well, locally advanced but also contained.

This apparent Bad News was different.

The thing is, I'd had a fall the day before, while awaiting my turn under the radiation gun, while undergoing 24/7 pumped chemo simultaneously. Fainted, actually. Crumpled against a wall, then down onto a tile floor. Then spent hours in the emergency room getting tested and interviewed and prepped for an unscheduled, unsettling session inside the MRI (magnetic resonance imaging) machine, all so that my medical team could have an updated picture of my compromised health status via a closer look at my brain. (*"Has it spread...?"* was thought but unsaid.)

But just before: Here comes Doc-in-Training...with my whole-body future in his hands...and he's read a report that said something about two spots in or on my skull. Seems he knows lots more than my wife and I do just now. And then he drops the Nuke about the bad news. Without first checking with his supervisors. Without any hint of seasoned bedside manner.

"Sorry about the bad news," he said, just once. But I kept hearing it over-and-over that morning, at least until we could talk with my radiation oncologist, the one who'd ordered the MRI the day before, the doctor whom I'd come to trust so far-so fast, because she didn't seem afraid of this whole diagnosis. She'd seemed confident enough that this cancer thing was corralled down below in my midsection. In my colon. More precisely: in my rectum. But that it hadn't spread. Still, protocol called on her to order the brain pictures, because, as a colleague explained: "We have to rule things out."

Her senior colleague also had said: Sometimes when you go looking around, with all the new equipment, you're bound to find something. Even if it's "just ditzels." Even if they may seem to be bad news when they aren't. Ditzels, it turns out, are stray matter, or shadows, or harmless scar tissue that may have come from a bump to the head 15 years ago. Or from a baseball that knocked me down with a concussion more than 30 years ago, back in my home town near Chicago. Main thing is, was: Ditzels, in context, aren't cancer. And so they may not be bad, or horrid, news.

Turns out the spots on my MRI were in fact mere ditzels. A doctor who did the reading of the images had diligently noted them on the report; and said they should be followed. But the doc did not say they were cancerous. Then the Saturday morning delivery guy bungled delivery of the news, assuming it was Bad when it wasn't (yet). Then we got another opinion. And I went on to have a couple of calm, reassuring discussions with my team of doctors about the false sense of alarm we'd all just lived through. Cancer care is not automatic.

I went back to my regularly scheduled program: chemo, radiation, hydration (more water—to help prevent future fainting spells caused by all this), the works. I went back older, wiser, and far-more schooled in the importance of getting a second, or a third opinion, no matter the cost or inconvenience.

And sometimes on an unscheduled, stop-in-your-tracks Saturday.

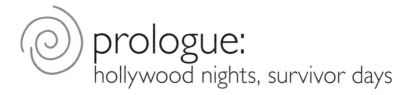

prologue:
hollywood nights, survivor days

The lights went down, and my heart-rate went up. But hold on, *thuh-thump, thuh-thump*: what the hell am I doing at the Academy Awards—*live in Los Angeles*—a guest at the (then-)Kodak Theatre, looking down at the unspooling of an Oscars telecast I won't ever forget? What am I doing in the third balcony—clad in a stiff tux with a crooked-cocked, bowtie—when I honestly thought, not so long ago, that the cancer I was fighting in my body might kill me? The short answer is, short answer was: I was rooting for my wife. This was Paula's moment, *maybe*, her time in the spotlight. Maybe even *Her Year*! And there I was, sitting in the nosebleed seats, while she and her three fellow filmmakers sat down below, way below, in the far-front Stage Left section of the orchestra, awaiting the callouts, the film clips, the search-and-find spotlights that possibly could mean that the woman who nursed me back to life from what felt like near-death from Stage 3 cancer was maybe now going to be called onto the biggest Stage in the world. To receive an award like no other.

And then the 1998 Oscar winner himself, Matt Damon, said, "And the Oscar goes to, *The Cove*!"

I remember jumping out of my seat and hugging my friend leaping next to me. Un*effing*believable. The little film that could.

My wife, the producer, now of an Oscar-winning film. My wife, who had held my hand in our seventh year of marriage when we walked into the underground radiation therapy room in San Francisco, pretending that things weren't really so awful. My wife, who shoved her hand under my skull after I had fainted and collapsed in a crumpled heap from dehydration-fatigue-undernutrition during chemo—and then exhorted the nearest doctor in the hallway to DO SOMETHING! Now my wife, a producer on the 2009 documentary, *The Cove*, was heading up to the Stage with the director and two of her fellow filmmakers to accept the award for Best Documentary Feature. The Best. She was, she is. I dedicate *My Cancer Year* to My Amazing Wife. What she did for me was no less amazing than what she did for the award-winning film. You could say, in more ways than one, that at times she saved us both.

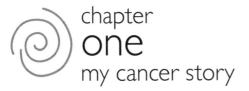

chapter
one
my cancer story

mad colon disease

At first, I thought it was the lousy British food. I had
landed in London in mid-June and succumbed to a
wicked case of jet jag. Or so I thought. A week, two, then
three went by, and still I wasn't sleeping through the night.
Restless; not in any pain, just not sleeping, and I hadn't been
eating all that well, either. "Bangers and mash, buddy?" Not
hardly.... My wife, Paula, and I had arrived in the UK last
summer, set to stay for the better part of a year. She would
serve as associate producer on the big *Harry Potter* film; I'd write
from overseas, traveling back and forth to the States when necessary for work.... After a month or so, my sleep still somewhat restless, I notice I've lost some weight. Chris Columbus, the director
[*Home Alone, Stepmom*] and longtime friend of mine and my wife,
asks Paula one day at dinner if I'm okay; he sees I've lost weight,
too. I also start to feel occasional cramps in my stomach, or lower,
even, down toward my groin. Upwards of my perineum, maybe,
somewhere deep down there...I also have diarrhea at least a couple
of times a week (British toilet paper sucks, by the way—c'mon, the
war's been over 55 years), which I attribute to not only the plebian

British food but to the pints of warm ale that I'm trying to get used to, nightly, at the local Haverstock Arms pub.

No health ignoramus, I decide to call a doctor in London to see if what I have is a flare-up of colitis, the disease I was diagnosed with—and treated for—back in New York in 1982. I find a doc fairly easily at the Wellington Hospital, which in the two-tiered health-care system in England seems to me to treat the moneyed tier...(tea and biscuits in the lobby while we wait).

Dr. Wong takes my history and nods his head at the suggestion of colitis. Then he ushers me into the room next door. Quite polite, he asks if he can "perform" a digital rectal exam. (I assume he means on my rectum.) I say fine. And so he does, quickly. And as he removes his gloved finger, we both notice traces of blood. He asks (again politely) if he thinks we should do a flexible sigmoidoscopy—scope my large intestine—and I think not. I'll get that done back in the States, I say. And I'll be home for a week next month.... I get a prescription for some hydrocortisone foam (in other words, an uninviting suppository), which, he says, should help in the meantime.... (He doesn't ask, politely, to insert the first dose.)

Looking back, I can say that both Dr. Wong and I get home that night thinking I have a case of colitis. Turns out we were wrong. We've all heard of mad cow disease—mad colon disease, maybe?

the diagnosis [part I]

INTERIOR: Master bedroom of our Boulder, Colorado, home, focus on phone on nightstand next to bed.

EXTERIOR: Wickedly bright sunshine, some clouds over the Flatirons and foothills.

CUE SOUND: Phone rings.

"Hello."

"Mr. Pesmen?"

"Yes..."

This is my doctor, my gastroenterologist, I can tell, on the line.

"Mr. Pesmen..." (Uh-oh, he's said my name twice in five seconds; not a good sign when you've been waiting for five hours for a phone call from someone who has been waiting for results from the pathology lab....)

"I've got some bad news..."

SYNOPSIS: This is no screenplay; this is not the theater. This is (my) real life. It has just been threatened....

skating away [part I]

For some reason, after I hang up with the doctor, I decide to go ahead and go ice-skating, just like I'd planned, with my friend Tom and his daughter in downtown Boulder. Call it denial, shock, incomprehension. For now, I still feel strong, I don't want to call or talk to anyone.... Paula isn't home...maybe being on the ice will somehow soothe me. I am lost, but head downtown with my skates in my hands. I park the car, lock up, and hear tinny speakers blaring "Jingle Bells." Three days till Christmas....

the diagnosis [part II]

SCENE: Master bedroom, still.

"It turns out they found some cancer cells in there," the doctor says of the pathologist. *"I am really sorry."*

I am stunned but do not cry. Instead, my body convulses slightly. Sitting on my bed, hunched over the phone, I feel as if I've just been in a minor car wreck...but all's...almost...okay.

My journalistic instincts take over and I start taking notes furiously..."adenocarcinoma...second opinion...final pathology report after the weekend...need to get you to a good surgeon... don't know the stage yet...after surgery you'll know more... really sorry to give you this news...."

Merry Christmas.

SYNOPSIS: Forget the car wreck. Feels like I have been hit by a train and have entered another world. I am now a cancer patient. December 22, 2000.

skating away [part II]: my secret

For an hour and 15 minutes, I don't tell a soul. I skate and make small talk, waiting for 4:00 to arrive, when I'm supposed to pick up Paula at a friend's. She knows we've been waiting for the call and, as soon as she hops in the car, asks me if I've heard anything. I lie and say no. My secret for 10 more minutes. I don't want to tell her until we get home. I feel like an ass lying to my wife about something so important, but I tell myself I'm doing it for her comfort.

When I tell her, we're in the kitchen, seated at the kitchen table.

"Paula," I say, "the doctor did call." Pause. She looks at me as if she is extremely hungry, though I know it is a look of fear.

"What? What?"

"I have cancer," I say. And nothing more.

She starts breathing heavily, then starts to shake. She starts to cry, I don't yet, then can't help but join her. Then she says she has to get down on the floor, right here, right now, or else she may faint.

My wife is now flat on her back on our white-tiled kitchen floor; we are both crying-heaving-crying, and I cradle her head in my hands and tell her to keep breathing.

"It's going to be okay," I say, not knowing if it will.

My wife and I both are now on the kitchen floor, letting this news sink in.

the diagnosis [part III]

SCENE: Downtown Denver, four-story medical building.

INTERIOR: Surgeon's office.

"You have rectal cancer, a kind of colon cancer," Doctor Second Opinion says. A weird dude to my eyes, kind of jumpy and unsettled, this over-eager surgeon has a good reputation among his peers. Plus he's one of the few docs we were able to see over the holidays…. Weird Dude Doc, after doing a rectal exam, then sits me in another room and compares my tumor to a rather large, gnarly bonsai tree that's thriving in a pot on his windowsill. He starts talking about growth, and I'm not liking this analogy at all. *"This man will not operate on me,"* I think as I take copious notes, realizing that surgeons' skill has little to do with their personalities.

CUT TO: The University of Colorado Health Sciences Center.

INTERIOR: Exam room of Dr. Third Opinion, Robert McIntyre, M.D.

"I agree you have rectal cancer," Dr. McIntyre of the University of Colorado says. *"The question is how much of the colon will we have to remove…."* I like this guy, his manner, his calm demeanor, his apparent mastery of the diagnosis with only limited information, which is why he's prepping me for a series of CT scans later this day, ordered by Dr. Cory Sperry, a friend of ours and a friend of his, to see if any cancer has spread to my lungs, abdomen, or liver…. This guy could operate on me, I think. And after he calls two days later to tell us the CT scans look *"good…I see the tumor, but the lungs, abdomen, and liver look clear,"* Paula and I feel like we've been given a reprieve. Good doc. Good results following a horrifying few days, and aftershock. Now, maybe, we can set up a plan to kick this cancer's ass, to turn perhaps the wrong phrase….

SYNOPSIS: I try to focus on some of Doc McIntyre's last words to Paula and me as we huddled in the exam room: *"Cancer is a word, not a sentence."* I'm curable.

tough call

Waiting. And wondering why I'm sitting on my bed on Saturday morning, delaying the inevitable. Waiting to call my family in Chicago and tell them the news. Making the wrong call and the right call at the same time, deciding to start by calling my sister, Beth. After all, she's my only sibling, just a couple of years older, 45, and has been through a major assault, having lost her first husband, Art, to leukemia when he was 35 and she was 32, a rock then; I expect her to be a rock now.

"I have cancer," I blurt after we chat about who-in-the-hell-remembers for about a minute. A slight pause. Longer pause, then a mournful wail and sob and heaving of breath and sound and emotion I have never heard emanate from my sister. Or from anyone close to me. Positively frightening. I'm now shaking, taking this in, realizing that maybe I've touched a dormant nerve that reached right back to that day when she became a widow, in July 1988.

Haunting, her sobs. "No! *Noooooooooo, noooo!*" And then she recovers. And then we settle into the shaken rhythms of our breathing, somehow feeling stronger, if only for a minute. I grab Paula's hand a little tighter while we buck up and prepare for The Next Call.

At 69 and 72, my mom and dad, Sandy and Hal, are to me a model couple. Semi-retired, semi-hip (my mom can still get away with leather pants; my dad, a leather bomber jacket), semi-serious about fitness, and married happily for nearly all of their 49 years together. I've got to "protect" them but can't delay any longer.

"I'm okay," I tell my mother as she asks, rhetorically, how I am. A signal from son to mother. She knows "okay" means something's wrong, though she turns out to be a rock. "I have cancer," I choke out to her, wondering if the fact that her mom died of cancer at 41, when she was only nine, has somehow steeled her against some of the worst medical news she could hear. My dad is a different story. He takes in the diagnosis, breaks up, then says, "You...have my colon." He repeats it. I'm confused, as my father has never had intestinal problems. He hands the phone off to my mom, shaken, and she tells me we will get through this and come out the other side....

Weeks later, I learn what my father was trying to tell me through emotional upheaval: "You can *have* my colon." At a literal loss for words, he was telling me he was willing to donate his, or part of his, large intestine to me, no matter how unlikely a scenario this could ever be. I'm glad I didn't know what he meant at the time.

not home alone

After Paula e-mails Chris Columbus and a few other people she's working with on the Potter movie, Chris calls our home immediately. He has put in calls to friends, including Robin and Marsha Williams, in San Francisco, to try to help us get fourth or fifth opinions at University of California, San Francisco, a top cancer center and the one that the Columbuses and Williamses have the utmost trust in.... It's also the hospital where Paula has some strong contacts, from years of helping coordinate movie screenings and benefits that have aided UCSF fundraising.

Almost unbelievably, Chris and his wife, Monica Devereux, immediately offer us the use of their home in San Francisco if we should choose to go there for treatment. And within hours, Marsha

Williams is on the phone with Paula...then me...talking about how important it is to get the best doctors for cancer treatment...and that she knows how to help us find them at UCSF. An unlikely Hollywood connection to my cancer, I am thinking, but there is friendship at the core of these gestures, not glamour or glitz. I am amazed at the outreach that's seemingly coming into our world, one call at a time....

happy frickin' birthday

Lashing out at Doctor Worthless in our darkened bedroom back in Boulder. We're home, "relaxing" and packing, getting used to powerful pain meds (and stool softeners to counteract their constipatory effects), and I'm still angry, I realize through late-night sobbing, at the Denver doctor who shall remain nameless, for now, who calls himself a gastroenterologist but did not, four to five months ago (*after* Dr. Wong's bloody finger and recommendation of a sigmoidoscopy), perform even a digital rectal exam that should have discovered this two-inch-long "locally invasive" tumor. Laziness? Maybe. HMO pressures to see too many patients per hour? Doubt It. The worthless doc didn't see fit to look where he should have, when he should have, as most competent gastroenterologists would suggest. I stop crying, settle down for a long fight, and try to find grace in this situation on a day that is probably the worst birthday my wife Paula has ever endured.

I'm prone most of the day and unable to get to the store to buy a card or present for my partner, the love of my life, who cries as I present her, shortly after midnight, with a 39th-birthday card with 39 hand-drawn hearts that I've fashioned from a folded business card of mine, drawing and writing in the bathroom between our two sinks. Happy frickin' birthday indeed.

future best-seller?

My best friend, Geoff, whom I've known since 1970, calls from Chicago: "I got an idea," he says. "You can do a book, call it: *Me, Cancer, and Geoff.* Instead of a book about how you and your wife got through this together, it'll be a buddy book about how I helped you kick cancer. I'll be calling you every day; people aren't expecting that." Pause. "You're sick," I say. "I know," he says. "But I gotta ask you: Does this mean I'll have to do one of those Run-Walk things with you in five years?"

the diagnosis [part IV]

SCENE: Exterior, UCSF Surgery Faculty Practice Building, 400 Parnassus Avenue, San-Francisco.

INTERIOR: Office of Dr. Mark Lane Welton, colorectal surgeon.

"...I believe your case is not a slam dunk; but I don't think it's one of my 14-hour operations, either," Dr. Welton says in the first hour of our meeting. *"It's probably a three-to four-hour operation."*

We soon learn that the cancer was found very late.

"Your cancer is advanced," Dr. Welton tells us.

"Then why didn't they find it in my screening three years ago?" I snap.

Dr. Welton shakes his head and tells me, *"I'd guess it's at least five years old."*

SYNOPSIS: He seems confident surgery will cure me, but he won't openly rip his colleagues. (Seems he believes Dr. Worthless and other private-practice gastros aren't as adept in colonoscopy as many practicing docs at university med centers, such as UCSF.) I like his style and honesty. If I have to be cut up, I want Dr. Welton to do the job.

probing my nodes

Lying on my back, waiting for doctor whomever from UCSF "paths" (pathology) to enter the room to do an FNA (fine-needle aspiration) of my inguinal lymph nodes, down by the groin and perineum, where the body normally doesn't invite needles in... poke, dig, poke, dig, poke, dig, he does. All negative—great! No cancer cells found. But he has to probe each one again, he tells me, a second time, to be "more sure."

Great, I'm thinking, and Dr. Daphne Haas-Kogan is still planning to zap my nodes, anyway, with God knows how many radiative "grey," for good measure, I later learn…. Gotta rush so the next docs can operate on me and insert a chemotherapy "port" in my chest…then Paula's gotta toss me on a United plane and fly my ass home for the weekend. Looks like we've made the choice: San Francisco for my treatment and surgery; back home to Colorado for the healing.

the team

Learning, in a hurry, that when you have cancer you don't have just one doctor. In my case, my team includes:

◎ Alan Venook, M.D., medical oncologist, UCSF

◎ Mark Lane Welton, M.D., colorectal surgeon, UCSF

◎ Daphne Haas-Kogan, M.D., radiation oncologist, UCSF

◎ Jonathan Terdiman, M.D., gastroenterologist, UCSF

◎ Jerry Ashem, nurse, home chemotherapy provider, Life Care Solutions

◎ Nancy Rao, N.D., naturopath and acupuncturist, Boulder,
Colorado

◎ Paula Dupré Pesmen, associate producer, wife, partner

eight words you don't want to hear

It's something I won't soon forget...there I am, splayed out on a
hard exam table in the radiation-therapy room, hospital PJ bottoms
pulled halfway down my crotch...when a senior member of the rad/
oncology team addresses a younger doctor after viewing my simulation—the precise position I will be in when radiation beams will
enter my body. He uses eight words: "The penis is going to have
a reaction." In other words, the penis (which would be mine) will
very likely develop a sunburn of sorts, perhaps over six weeks of
absorbing nearby radiation waves. Note to self: "Prepare."

treatment: chemotherapy

Surprise: In this new new age of personal electronics, it appears
that my six weeks of chemotherapy will be administered by a
machine, not a person.

Small enough to fit in a fanny pack, BlackBerryish in person-
ality, the portable pump I name Abbott, built by Abbott Labs
outside Chicago, will be in charge of delivering a toxic chemical,
a toxic cancer-fighting chemical, 5-fluorouracil, into my blood-
stream. (I could opt for weekly visits to an infusion center, where
my medical oncologist has his office, but since I'm on a low-dose
regimen, Abbott seems the way to go.) He's got a small screen,
24 buttons, lots of chirps and beeps, and a clear plastic tether tube
that stretches about four-and-a-half feet.

Once a week, a home nurse will come and change the medicine, flush my "line," take my blood pressure, draw some blood,
change his gloves, don a mask, change the needle that fits in the port

inside my chest, swab the whole upper-right quadrant of chest with antiseptic, then tape me down, making me water-resistant, not quite waterproof, for at least six weeks. More chemo later? I wonder.... Yes, I learn soon enough, but it probably won't be porta-pumped in.

treatment: radiation

Beep. Beep. Beep. Beep.

Whirr. Whirr.

Bzzzzz. Bzzzzz. Bzzzzz...Silence.

Ker- CHUNK....

Welcome to the world of Radiation Oncology, Day One of the six-week treatment, as part of a protocol that's not practiced every-where. Some docs say, till more data are in, the tumors should be taken surgically first, followed by chemo and radiation. But not the docs we have on our team. It's a sandwich kind of cancer-fighting. BEEP/WHIRR, then surgery; then chemo afterward, as necessary.

Today, in the basement of UCSF's Long Hospital, amid the city's first big storm of the year, I try to find a quiet moment as the Big Gun goes off. *Beep, Beep, Beep. Whirrr...Bzzzz....*

my 24/7/6 anti-cancer machine

Wondering why some people are so afraid to use the word "cancer" when they e-mail or write notes to me sending warm thoughts.... Thanking the literary lords that a 10-year-old daughter of one of my friends sent a card that said, up front: "Dear Curt, I hope you fight off your cancer.... Love, Rebecca"

How the hell can you take this sucker on...if you can't call it by its name? It's cancer, and I'm hooked up to a porta-chemo-pump stashed in a fanny pack that's "pre-treating" my tumor while I get daily blasts of radiation (weekends off), courtesy of the GE Clinic

2300 radio-therapy accelerator. I'm a 24/7/6 (six months total treatment) anti-cancer assault unit, with all this technology comin' at me, going in me, going through me and God knows where else into the walls of the underground radiation oncology unit named for Walter Haas, the Levi Strauss magnate, and dedicated in 1983.

Otherwise, it's January 2001, and, shoot, things are great.

eat more, weigh less

Weighing in one afternoon while in treatment at 168. Wondering where the pounds went so quickly. I was 183 before I left for England last summer. My appetite is down, so is my general attitude toward eating. "Food is no longer for pleasure," Dr. Haas-Kogan ("Call me Daphne") says. "It's your job."

sex and my cancer [part I]

Haven't found lots of info on the standard patient Websites about sex and colon cancer.... Here's what I know so far: In one month of being a colon-cancer patient, I've had sex twice, once what I would term successfully. The other time, well, that's what I know about sex and my cancer.

happy anniversary

One month after the diagnosis. My anger has dissipated toward my doofus doctor who never stuck his middle finger up my anus all fall 2000, while I complained of rectal pain—it's right there in his carefully written notes in the records I snatched, or rather requested, from his office. I mean, of course my anger has cooled....

Consider: A patient at higher-than-average risk of colon cancer comes in and complains of stomach pain, rectal pain, and diarrhea (some would call that "a change in bowel habits..."), and in your wisdom you decide not to perform a basic digital rectal exam. Cruel irony, perhaps, that the cancer you'd later find would show up in the rectum. And was, other surgeons have said, large enough to have been felt by a doctor's finger.... And if you had glanced through my records, you would have seen that you performed a screening colonoscopy on me a few years ago, and that I had some suspect tissue that turned out to be benign. No need to check back, I guess. I know how hard doctors have to work these days.

Four or five months earlier, diagnosis would only mean I'd be a lot more comfortable right now and have a better—as hard as it is to say—chance of cure, whatever that means in oncological parlance. You can have your five-year survival rates, Dr. Worthless. You've called me exactly once in a month's time to check on me, your patient that you recently diagnosed as having colon cancer. Remember me? Happy frickin' anniversary. Maybe see you in court.

"a possibly fatal event"

Guinea-pig Friday. Seven hours of waiting for a cautionary scan of my lungs and legs, all because I reported having shortness of breath this morning and my surgeon, Dr. Welton, and his resident scrunched their eyebrows like squirrels (if I'm a guinea pig, they're squirrels) and thought of the remote possibility of PE—pulmonary embolism—"a possibly fatal event."

I have a few risk factors, you see: an open line running into my veins for chemo; I have cancer; I am over 40 years old; have an infection; and have been largely immobile. Better safe than dead, they think but don't say. (Reportedly, it's one of the most frequently missed diagnoses in medicine.) So there goes our Friday afternoon and evening. We wait, and wait, for a space in the CT queue...and Doc Daphne comes over from the hospital next door to try to help move things along...at 8:00 p.m. on a Friday night. Three kids she has at home, and she's with Paula and me. This is what you call care.

This is what leads to Paula getting for her four Harry Potter T-shirts from her stash in London. My lungs and legs turn out to be clear.

a sob story

Waking up with bad chemo/radiation nausea and diarrhea... an hour on the john to start the day...followed by 30 minutes of intense sobbing in bed, broken occasionally by heavy breathing (to relax me), the tears flow and I plead for "a break." I know part of this frustration is from yesterday's seven hours of helplessness and waiting for exams...and the possibility of "a fatal event," as if colorectal cancer isn't a possibly fatal event. I begin to view crying as part of healing. It's probably in the cancer-support books that the nurses gave me and that I've yet to read.... Fourth, you cry.

lick me

After too many days of chemo/poison pumping through my veins, my body sends its first signal of being pissed off at the assault—a rash, or rawness, on the back and center of my tongue, all raised and ugly, what the doctor calls "mucositis"; what a nurse says might be thrush...we'll worry about it tomorrow. Today, I'll just add some antibiotics to my arsenal to try and hit the elusive fever that kicks up each afternoon and evening, from 99.4 to 100.5 or so, possibly related to last week's discovery of an abscess. "Possibly," say Dr. Daphne and Dr. Welton. Lotsa *possiblys* in this long-term anti-cancer contest that's still in the early stages. Even a temporary alarm set off by Abbott—signaling occlusion in the tubes that send 5-FU chemo drug into my body—doesn't trip us up for long.

An 800 number, plus a knowing pharmacist on the "home health care/Life Care Solutions" hotline, helps us get Abbott back on track with only a 10-minute interruption in cancer-kick-butt service. With *ER* playing in the background on TV, my little chemo emergency couldn't have asked for a more macabre backdrop. Blood and guts all over the Mitsubishi big-screen TV...a portable-CD-player-sized pump in my hands, sending peeling alarm signals and not responding to my attempted repair. And I can't very well call Dr. Greene.

i don't like mondays

Setting the alarm for 8:45 a.m., which to the rest of the world sounds late, I know, but for someone who is woken up every two hours to take a piss because radiation waves have riled up my bladder tissue till it's as angry as an 84-year-old's who's got a mean case of prostatitis...truth is, I don't want to arise at 8:45. I could easily sleep till 10:00, since I haven't enjoyed real REM-type sleep for what seems like a week.

Waiting for nurse Jerry, all earnest and bearded and careful and responsible-like, to come visit and slip on the rubber gloves and rip a bent needle out of the port that's been surgically implanted in my chest...new week, new bag of "dope" for my main man, Abbott.... It's all good, I suppose, but I don't enjoy lying flat on my back with anti-splash pads beneath my chest and torso. (Chemo is poison, let's remember; we don't want that stuff splashing about the linens, much less our respective skins....)

Mondays mean a whole week ahead of whomping the bad cells with good X-rays and 168 milliliters of 5-fluorouracil cocktail, my chemo drug of choice...so by Friday night or Saturday morning, I will almost certainly feel like shit. Which means, they tell me, Mondays should actually be "good" days, because I've had the weekend off from the radiation assault...and my body's had a chance to "recover."

Shoot, other than that, Mondays are fine specimens of the week. When you're normal, that is. When you're Cancer Boy, you're just a bit more skeptical about this fine day....

bonding

Flipping off a friend, in a good way, a male-bonding way, as I lie on the couch, fatigued and diseased. He's flown 25 hundred miles to visit me, my old roommate Todd, and at one point I look over at him in the living room, our eyes meet, and I give him the finger. He understands completely. What men want. A tough way to say, "Thanks for leaving your job and family for a few days to come hang with me as I get chemo'd and radiated." A guy thing. I love the guy. He's here. I'm hurtin'. So "Flip off." Makes perfect sense, as Paula wonders, maybe, what in the hell I've just done to my friend. She understands, maybe not completely.

can cancer be embarrassing?

An East Coast friend, whom I've known since 1980, calls: "So...it must be hard having cancer in a place that's embarrassing?"

I pause, weighing the absurdity of the comment, then respond.

"I guess so. But I guess I'd rather have colon cancer than brain cancer." Insensitive dude, I am as well, knowing that I disrobe every day in the bowels of UCSF's Long Hospital alongside patients who are being treated radiotherapeutically for cancer in and on their brains.

That's not so embarrassing? I wonder. And we go on to talk about, believe it or not, the New York Yankees.

sunburn where the sun don't shine

"It's gonna get worse before it gets better;" says Doc Daphne as I hit the home stretch of "Intro to Radiation 101" (six-week course). Sunburnlike burns on my inner buttocks, burned and raw skin where groin meets thigh, and, yes, a scorched penis. Time to learn, from the radiation nurse, how to use and apply the wickedly priced, aloe-based ointment known as: Carrington RadiaCare Gel

Hydrogel Wound Dressing. It's soothing, I soon find, as I hitch up my drawers and shuffle off after getting dressed, holding my wife's left hand in my right.

getting to know pain

Don't know why I'm surprised, five weeks into treatment, how much cancer hurts, but I am. The pain I've gotten to know, that renders me horizontal at least five hours a day, has started messing with my mind. I've been hurting at least four months now. Even with narcotics (and I have good ones), I hurt more profoundly, more often, than I can take. It is so deep inside, it actually radiates from my pelvis out into my legs and down to the soles of my feet. It gets to where I start naming the types of pain: stabbers, daggers, and achers. (Achers hurt the worst.)

Driven to the couch two/three times a day, I wonder what it would take to become part of California's legal medical-marijuana program. The docs at UCSF don't seem all that familiar with it, but they give time four phone numbers to try and a list of instructions. Gotta check this out further.

down for the count

Whipping around the corner in Long Hospital's basement, late for my daily beams of radiation, scurrying into the men's changing room (does it *really* matter whether you wear hospital gowns and pajama bottoms instead of T-shirts and jeans when it's radiation we're talking about?), and getting undressed/dressed in almost record time....

Feeling light-headed as I wait for my appointed slot under The Gun, looking for an empty chair—"Do you want me to get you a chair?" my sister Beth says—and I say no, feeling macho, but also feeling more lightheaded than I know—*slam/crumple/thump*—I'm down on the tile floor in an instant—unconscious. Ten seconds, 20, maybe 30. When I come to, I see three sets of eyes staring down at me.... "Curt, Curt, can you hear me?" my wife, Paula, pleads. "I need a gurney and a pulse ox!" Doc Daphne shouts, *ER*-style. I am coming to...quickly...not knowing why I went down or what my elbow hit on the way down, 'cause it's hurting but not bleeding, and suddenly there are eight people hovering around me on my gurney as I "stabilize."

Wheeling me into the Rad Room, the radiation therapists ask me if I can stand. I say yes, not knowing if I can and yet not knowing that I had the beginnings of a seizure while on the ground. I quickly learn that radiation treatments *don't stop*...just 'cause a patient goes down.

Rolling into the ER upstairs moments later, I'm wired for an EKG to check my heart, and the battery of tests commences... blood, urine, neuro, orthostatics [blood pressure standing and sitting]. Bottom line, the docs think I've been dehydrated due to the chemo and other aspects of cancer treatment; and my red-blood-cell count is low.

The assault continues, as Doc Daphne checks in before my discharge to suggest that we do "a head MRI" sometime soon...takes a while for my brain to click in...she's checking for balance problems...or maybe a blood clot caused my fainting spell?...or else, well, maybe she's just gonna scan my head, MRI-style, to rule out that slim chance that I have cancer in my brain. The assault continues....

showerdance

With a [chemo port] line going into my chest, with a four-inch-by-four-inch swatch of Tegaderm breathable-but-not-waterproof bandage on top of the contraption, I'm not allowed to take showers as I used to, before I became a cancer patient.

I wash my hair in the sink (using a plastic Pac Bell Park cup for the big-rinse finish) most days or do a quick, body-turn shower, wherein I leave my chemotherapy pump parked in its fanny pack just outside the shower door and wet what I can, soap what I can, then washcloth the rest, once I've successfully rinsed, keeping my trusty chemo pump, "Abbott," dry.

we got game

Walking across the street, trailing my nephew Clark, who's come to visit and, frankly, is hoping to play some hoop with his uncle. His *fatigued* uncle.

He dribbles, shoots, scores, so do I! He spins the red-and-black Harlem Globetrotter promotional basketball lazily, woozily, on his right middle finger. I catch the ball and show Clark how to spin it faster and how to get the ball to spin on my/his finger for 10 seconds instead of five....

Shots go in; three-pointers clang off the rim; Paula shoots her first shot and somehow gets it stuck—lodged—between the rim brace and the backboard. I struggle to jog/run after rebounds...I'm huffing...but fact is...80 days after my diagnosis, I am once again playing an outdoor game.

sex and my cancer [part II]

Wondering, in bed, how long it will take for the barbecued, irradiated skin on my package to return to normal color and texture.... Finding that having an erection and doing something pleasurable with it hurts in such odd, frightening ways in the first weeks after radiation treatment...that it makes you think twice about having an erection and doing something pleasurable with it.

leave your dignity at the door

"Tough-ass Sim," is all I can say...and it's not a sorry pun. It's a day of Radiation Simulation I'll remember as one of the worst, particular to my type of colorectal cancer, to my type of pre-surgery treatment.

"Curt, you may have to leave your dignity at the door," says Doc Daphne as she leads me to a treatment room. Within minutes, I am bottomless, on my belly, on a hard table, with doctors and therapists around me, drawing Magic Marker targets on my ass and hips, calling out measurements that I don't understand. The rectal/anal probes that irritate tumor tissue I do understand. Quickly. I groan like a farm animal. This is what the good doctor meant by leaving my dignity at the door. Feeling like a roasted pig with an apple in its snout: "Come get me—I'm done."

Forty-five minutes later, my pelvis is now prepped to guide the beams of my last few radiation "boosts." "I'm sorry," Doc Daphne says of The Sim. "I'm really sorry."

finding god [part I]

Realizing, on day 71 after diagnosis, in year 43 of my life, that I have never prayed as regularly before.

well runs dry

If it's emotional dehydration I'm worrying about, and I'm worrying about Paula's "well" often, I find a few answers in her journal:

> *Curt's been on chemo & radiation for weeks—he's doing okay,*
> *but he's sick and very tired and still has a fever every night. We're*
> *fighting to keep weight on him, literally. Each meal is a battle between*
> *me and a guy called Nausea. I am determined to win and I do,*
> *because losing means that I'm letting Curt down.*

Today I had a meltdown. I was lying on the bed crying like a two-year-old late for a nap. I have to tell Curt, I'm tired of being the bad guy. I represent the things that bring him discomfort: food, medicine, trips to the hospital. I ride his butt each day to take a pain pill, go for treatment, eat, eat, eat.... I want to hold him and kiss him and nurture him well, but those things are just a part of his wellness. He lost 6 pounds last week and the doctor's concerned. I have to keep him eating. He's having very serious surgery soon and needs to be strong.

Cancer is trying to come between us. Where I used to lay my head, now lies a chemo port sewn into his chest. Nausea and fever cause him to need space. I tell Curt I want to be small so I can curl up in his arms and feel him. This disease is trying to isolate Curt from people he loves. I won't let it happen. He takes me to the chair where we curl up and he holds me like I'm his wife and everything feels good again. Today we've won.

nice 'n' angry

Getting a bill from Dr. Worthless in Denver for services "rendered"...wondering if/or how much I should pay the doctor who I believe fouled up my diagnosis and treatment for months last fall. Knowing part of what I believe is supported by my medical records. I'm still furious he never did digital rectal exams when I went to see him—twice—complaining of rectal pain last fall. There was—and is—a tumor where he could have felt it.

Thinking back to what Dr. Haas-Kogan told me not long ago about my disease: "Don't give up your license to be angry. No 43-year-old man should have to go through what you're going through."

My "license to be angry." I hadn't thought of things this way. Now I do.

the facts

- Colorectal cancer is the second-leading cause of cancer-related death in the U.S. (Lung cancer is the first.)
- Approximately 50,000 deaths due to cancer in 2010 were due to colorectal cancer.
- About 90 percent of people diagnosed with colon cancer are over age 50.

High-risk factors include:

1 Family history
2 A diet low in fiber and high in fat (mostly from animal sources)
3 Personal history of colon polyps
4 Personal history of chronic inflammatory bowel disease, Crohn's disease, or ulcerative colitis. People suffering from Crohn's disease or ulcerative colitis for more than 20 years are at more than twice the risk for colorectal cancer than the average person their age.

Symptoms of colorectal cancer may include:

1 Rectal bleeding
2 Blood in the stool
3 A change in bowel habits
4 Abdominal, rectal, or liver pain
5 Feeling of fatigue, loss of weight, or decreased appetite.

Doctors recommend that all people over 50 receive some type of screening, at least an annual FOBT, or fecal occult blood test. The American College of Gastroenterology recommends that people over 50 receive a colonoscopy at least once every 10 years, as well as an FOBT and a flexible sigmoidoscopy once every five years.

Patients diagnosed with ulcerative colitis or Crohn's disease are at particularly high risk and should undergo colonoscopy at least once every two years.

a head case

Driving across town in early afternoon to the shiny, happy, new UCSF Cancer Center, to get my chemo line unhooked, to get the needle removed from the port in my chest, to get back to living without being tethered to a pump/fanny pack that even has to sleep with me under my pillow. Progress. I'm free, in a way, six weeks before surgery, but tonight I have a date with my wife, my friend Jim, and the MRI machine.

The docs, the good folks taking care of me, who haggled over my fainting spell last week, are going to have a close look at my brain. They want the MRI to "rule out" cancer in my brain as a cause.... Ten times louder (slo-mo jackhammers), three times more uncomfortable (claustrophobia) than the CT scans I now know too well...the MRI of the matter inside my skull comes out pretty well...at least for now.

Bottom line: no cancer found in my brain, but, and there's always a *but*, there are two fuzzy spots on the film outside my skull that the docs may want to take a closer look at. When you have cancer, there are sound reasons sometimes to keep looking for more cancer. This means for me another round of tests in the future, a round of tests that Paula and I don't want to deal with right now. My docs give me a break, at least for now.

the diagnosis [part V]

EXTERIOR: Master shot. Rolling clouds, west to east, across San Francisco Bay.

INTERIOR: Eighth-floor medical office, Moffitt Hospital, UCSF.

Meeting with my surgeon a month and a half before surgery, getting ready to schedule The Date, finding out I'll need at least three more scans and four more meetings with doctors before I get cut. Learning that I'll be losing most if not all of my colon in less than two months. Slipping into journalistic mode, I shut off emotions and hear "colostomy," "ileostomy"... bagged for life. Or for at least a long time.

SYNOPSIS: Major Lifestyle Change, a reasoned journalist might say, in exchange for Life.

finding god [part II]

Not realizing until my diagnosis, and until the news got out, how many friends and family members who never talk to me about religion regularly pray. Now they send word of including me in their nightly prayers and other prayer circles. A cousin of mine sends a miniature carving of a powerful-looking shaman...there's a guy I want to take into surgery with me.

heading home

Still reeling, and peeling, nine days after the last of the big radiation blasts...no more chemo pumping into my veins; wondering how long it takes to clear my body completely (if indeed it does clear completely).

Knowing I now have 3.3 weeks left to "heal" and get stronger back home in Boulder before the surgery; trying not to think about that right now...don't know that I could even handle the trip/airport/assholes—plus-three hours of sitting—just yet...popping a Vicodin to stifle the pain...taking a walk in the park, heavy legs and all, in Pac Heights to try and beat the fatigue.

But I don't. Beginning to understand why I saw that hospital flyer about a clinical study looking for subjects re: cancer fatigue. Fatigue is no small matter. No small malady. The sucker doesn't know when to leave. It is a key part of the assault.

I want, among other things, the lightness in my legs back.

high mileage/low mileage

Feeling like a low-mileage patient today...which means pretty good in cancer-doc speak. Hang around the oncology ward long enough and you'll hear hospital workers instantly, cruelly, assess new patients as "high mileage" or "low mileage." Which one's gonna take more work? Which one's got the better chance for cruising down the road, in years ahead?

Feeling like a human again...back home and healing after Round One of treatment. Walking slowly after lunch around the lake by our house, logging a total of 1.3 miles. High mileage, low mileage, whatever. It's actual miles, and I'm counting.

friends, finances, food

Settling back into our own home in Boulder after the two-month medical pilgrimage to San Francisco. Opening the first of the hospital bills with more zeros on the end than I can take seriously. Reconnecting with friends, who absolutely feel like family as they swarm the house in pre-ordained small-group waves...the first posse sneaking in the day before our arrival and stocking the house with food.

Second wave cooks us a Saturday-night turkey-meatloaf-mashed-pots-and-gravy dinner; third wave brings over take-out Chinese...which is all good, all fine, all warm and fuzzy-like...except that in my case, food that = love also = pain—almost instant pain after eating—and that reminds me I still have an angry, invasive adenocarcinoma residing at the end of my digestive tract.

dead man sleeping

Trying not to think about surgery, cancer, recovery, chemo, and going back to UCSF in three weeks. Luxuriating, almost, with

Paula's fresh soups, French-toast-with-strawberry breakfasts, late-night shakes to put the weight back on...and small groups of friends stopping by to check in, check on me, see how Paula's holding up....

Then a call comes, less than a week since we've been home. Her dog, our dog, Toto, the 13-year-old Maltese, died last night while asleep under the bed of Paula's mom in California, where he's been living for the past six months. No ordinary hound, Toto the Wonderdog. Can't help but weep through the late morning... what lousy timing. Then comes an unlikely knock on our door from a Boulder cop. Asks to come in, leads us to our living-room window, explaining that he is looking for clues.... Seems a dead man was found a few hundred yards from our house, in the 6.2 acres deemed "open space" by the city.... Whether the man was murdered or died-in-his-sleep we do not know. Cop doesn't, either, or at least he's not saying. I'm hurting, pelvically, colonically, taking this all in, trying to be strong on my feet, telling Officer Navarro that I was up between 3:40 and 5:00 a.m., in bed, and didn't hear anything. We didn't do it, officer. Now can you leave us to ponder... two deaths...too close to home...while I, we, just try to recover in "paradise"?

sex and my cancer [part III]

A wife (that would be mine) writes in her journal: "It's our 7th anniversary. I asked Curt if he had the seven-year itch. He said, 'only where the radiation burns are healing.' (That would be his groin, and that would be a 'no' to my question.)"

friendly fire

Walking toward Wonderland Lake, looking for the soccer field where my friend Tom is coaching his daughter and other seven-or-eight-year-olds. Hanging around with the parents, reminding myself that Paula and I aren't parents yet, and at 39 and 43, time is running short....

Wondering why I can't remember whether—at week 10 of my treatment—my sperm could ever recover and (safely) father a baby after all the radiation my groin, pelvis, and balls have been through. Thinking back to the day weeks ago when I banked sperm in that horrible windowless room in a San Francisco fertility clinic, just in case friendly fire of any sort would hurt our chances.

gotta have faith

Taking a walk to boost my strength from radiation and chemo, still not quite 170 pounds. Trying not to think too much about the surgery in two weeks, but how much is too much? I can't help but think—and say to Paula—"Do you realize we've trusted these doctors to leave my cancer inside me for three months?" (So they could treat it before surgery, instead of just cutting it out like some hospitals would have.) Once we signed on at UCSF, we learned about a new kind of faith. And fear.

true confession

ME: *"Hmmmmm...muhhhhh..."*

PAULA: *"You in pain?"*

ME: *"No."*

Pause.

ME: *"Hmmmmm...muhhhhh..."*

PAULA: *"You in denial?"*

ME: *"I guess so."*

golf and my cancer

Getting out of the house, putting and pitching in some cool, gray spring air at Flatirons Golf Course. Betting Jim a dollar-a-hole for closest-to-the-pin on the putting green, then swinging away, sort of, at a 75-yard target with a pitching wedge, aiming at a swalelike area littered with range balls.

Taking care not to take a full swing, else I may rip my implanted chest port and vein tube from their anchors under my skin by my right shoulder. Not sure whom to ask about golfing-with-a-chemo-port...knowing that a wicked swing might send me to a hospital for unscheduled surgery.... Kinda takes the sweetness out of the short shots that I hit rather well this day.

fear at thirty-five thousand feet

Trying to forget about my disease for a few more hours as we pack up and head back to San Francisco. A week of tests, then surgery. As we hit max altitude, I pick *Parade* out of the Sunday paper and unfortunately find a story by Tad Szulc, 74...a journalist who just happens to have colon cancer...that has spread unpredictably to his liver and lungs two years after surgery. "It's incurable," he writes. At this moment I am not afraid of the plane crashing. [*Editor's note: Szulc died shortly after the* Parade *story ran.*]

world spinning round

"I saw a lot of things spinning around my head this week," I tell Paula, trying to explain the feelings I have after yesterday's pelvic MRI, while lying on my back on a slab of hard plastic and foam, being slid, mechanically, into a chamberlike futuristic body scan, only it's not futuristic, it's now, CT-style, with unknown imaging parts spinning, whirring, racing around my body inside the machine, gaining speed and making magnetic pictures of body parts, body cavities, body systems from head to groin. And as the spin spins, a Teutonic male voice occasionally commands, and does so creepily, "Breathe in," "Hold" (for 16 seconds yet...), "Breathe out." And again. And again. It's all prep for surgery. It's new mapping for the docs to compare with the scans they took back in January. I'm spun out.

karma waves

Waiting for Doc Daphne, the radiation doc, in Exam Room 7 of Long Hospital's basement, who's left to read the whole batch of my new films, the ones that will say how well, or not, my treatment has been going...just me and Paula sitting in the room around lunchtime with the door closed, not thinking about lunch. For what if the tumor grew during my weeks at home?

"I wish I had your karma," Doc Daphne finally says after eyeing my CTs and taking a seat next to me. Good news again; all the tests show the tumor has either shrunk or not spread. This on the very day the City of San Francisco's department of public health issues me an official plastic-coated "Medical Cannabis Voluntary ID Program" card, which will enable me to buy marijuana for medicinal uses for up to one year from today. Twenty-five dollars it cost me, plus 25 for Paula's card, as "caregiver," who can get the drugs if I'm laid up...or retching from chemo that's ahead. And from what I learn about the surgery today...it's going to mean laid up, or down, for at least six weeks. Bit more karma, please?

sex and my cancer [part IV]

Taking a meeting I'd rather not take. Going to see Peter Carroll, M.D., chairman of the department of urology at UCSF, who's been asked to join my surgery team. "He's going to help me stay out of the prostate," Dr. Welton, my colorectal surgeon, says.

Stay out of the prostate indeed. It's not enough lousy luck that I— Mr. Health Book Author—get cancer, that I get colorectal cancer, that I'm going to have my abdominal organs rearranged: now one of the top urologic surgeons in the country tells me, after reviewing the MRI of my pelvis, that in surgery I may lose some of the nerves that help erections become erections. Without those nerves, bundled around the prostate and near the rectum, I understand in a hurry, I may soon be Viagra dependent, sexually speaking.

"We just want the cancer out," Paula tells Dr. Carroll. I think maybe we want a little more than that.

countdown

T minus 30 hours and counting...till they strip me, gown me, wheel me, scrub me, shave me, drug me, prep me, cut me, eviscerate me, probe me, stimulate me (erectile nerves, that is, using a newish procedure to try to save my sexual functions), reorganize me (turning my small intestines into my small-and-large intestines and anus...), de-cancer me, maybe "muscle-flap" me (as in plastic surgery if the surgical wound gets to be tricky to close), and bring me to, as a cancer patient, as a recovering colon-cancer patient who's going to be in pain and most likely minus one colon; they're gonna do all this and more in T minus 30 hours, and I wonder why a couple of friends have asked me quite recently, "Are you nervous?" What if I said, no, I wasn't? Thing of it is, I'm going in Tuesday morning, three months after my diagnosis, six weeks after my chemo/radiation regimen; I'm going in Tuesday morning, not nervous but frightened, to get a tumor out, God and all other higher powers willing.

the power of (legal) pot

Waking up one morning before dawn, with bone-numbing lower-body pain that starts me moaning-breathing-moaning and wakes up Paula. I get what the doctors mean when they say my tumor is low enough to be lodged in my pelvis. Time for narcotics, my man Vike [Vicodin], except it'll take 45 minutes to work. We both know that by now. Which is why we have four medical joints stashed in an Altoids tin box.

"Why don't you take some pot?" Paula says.

"It's too early," I tell her. "It's not even 6:15."

A beat, then Paula responds: "It's not like you're smoking it because you don't have a job!"

I light up. It works, masking the pain without making me high, till good brother Vike kicks in.

"play ball!"

You've got to give him points for trying. My surgeon, Dr. Welton, after meeting with Paula and me to have us sign consent forms and review next week's surgery, gives us a bit of consent, too. "We've got tickets to the Giants' Opening Day—but it's the day before surgery," Paula says. "Do you think it would be okay for Curt to go?"

"Yeah," he says, knowing full well I've got to be on a liquid diet all day and take major laxatives the night before the operation. "He should be fine. As a matter of fact, I think it would be good for you guys to go.

"You can think of it this way: Monday will be baseball Opening Day and Tuesday will be our Opening Day."

This I find almost funny.

night before

"It's gonna be okay," I say to Paula with eight hours to go till surgery.

Silence.

"You know why?" I ask.

She shakes her head no.

"Because of you, because of what I have to live for," I say.

Following chemo and radiation treatment, surgery was scheduled for April 3.

pre-op pep talk

"Hey," I say to Paula, after the travel alarm *chirps-chirps-chirps* us awake, "let's go get some cancer out." Sounds like I'm cheerleading on Surgery Day but I'm not. Just making light in the early-a.m. dark.

"Hey," I say, "let's go get some cancer out."

road trip

Rolling through the pitch-black streets of San Francisco toward the hospital, our pal Aimee at the wheel, Paula up front, me stretched out at an odd angle in between the backseat; still hurts to sit straight up on my tumor.

Time to cut the vile thing from my body. Traffic at 6:30's a breeze, though I'm wishing it weren't. I'm suddenly in no hurry... thinking about the odd positions they're gonna have me in throughout this ordeal...this total colectomy or whatever. Too late to worry, but I'm wondering, still, whether the pre-op chemo/ radiation combo actually shrank my tumor enough to allow these UCSF doctors to excise all of what we all want excised. Don't want to hear they got "most of it": that means I could be back here in a couple years, the "absolutely curable" me, rolling through the darkened streets once more, heading for more cancer surgery after having tried—and likely failed—to renew my six-year-old term life-insurance policy.

pre-op prep walk

As Dr. Mark Welton said last week, it's Opening Day! But before he opens me up and takes out what's evil, they've got to check me in, like at some hotel of horrors in the gloam of pre-sunrise, and they've got to have me perform a macabre march-of-the-day—with two other patients (one in a wheelchair) and a nurse in the lead, here we go!—from ground-floor check-in to pre-op anesthesia up on four.

Shuffling our way through the halls of Moffitt-Long Hospital, waiting for our appointed docs and drugs. Last time I'll be wearing street clothes for a week, I think, as I tote a large plastic "Patient Belongings" bag that now belongs to me. I look at Paula, who looks sad walking beside me; we're in the back of the pack....I feign a stop-look-and-run away from the group, like a kid on a fourth-grade field trip to some boring modern-art museum, only this ain't a museum and the only exhibit worth looking at around these parts is still lodged deep in my pelvis—call it Exhibit A. Or more accurately, Exhibit C.

cutting remarks

Can't say I saw what I'm about to say here, but if what they say is true about my operation, it didn't go well...it went better than well. I mean, "We got a better result than we even hoped for back in January," said Alan Venook, M.D., my medical oncologist. I'll take it.

I didn't see where the first scalpel started, but I do see I have an 11-inch abdominal incision, held closed by 42 metal staples, which artfully arcs around my belly button (doctors don't mess with belly buttons), where they "entered" and removed my entire colon and rectum (just lucky, I guess, as I've read 85 percent of colon-cancer patients don't need to have their entire colons removed—they just lose a few inches of intestine). I also feel but can't see a five-inch incision down around my anus, which means in order to excise my rectal tumor completely, they had to cut me from above and below. Not your standard, slam-dunk polyp removal, which is why the surgery took eight hours instead of two or three. [It was a stubborn rectal tumor, says Doc Welton, in retrospect. And it was, he reminds me: a newish, nerve-sparing operation... a TME, or total mesorectal excision, with which not all cancer surgeons are familiar.] There's also a newly created hole in my lower torso through which my intestines and stoma (aka my new anus) now feed.

And the good news again? Hey, they didn't need to use the fancified, intraoperative radiation machine that was on standby... and they didn't need to use the plastic surgeon to help "close" me. (He was on standby, too.) Final pathology says that the margins around the tumor were clear...which means my team done good. Very good. They grabbed 31 lymph nodes out of me, 30 of which were cancer-free. I'd be more worried about the one that wasn't, except that I now know at least a few other lymph nodes were probably also cancerous back in January and February...and my pre-op chemo/ radiation killed the cancer in those. Had they operated in January, I might've had six cancerous nodes and 25 "clean." So the single bad node doesn't worry me right now because, docs say, they got clear margins. The tumor and surrounding nodes were encapsulated. I can live with that, in more ways than one.

an ice place to visit

Welcome to the RR—recovery room—where they wheel me after the OR, where a lot happens in a hurry, in a flurry, and yet I remember only a few things:

1. that Paula was there to my right, telling me that "they...got...it...all";

2. that a nurse to my left, who was taking all sorts of measure-ments and checking multiple monitors and related tethers, had to leave in a hurry because her car was parked at a meter;

3. that I could...barely...breathe—felt like my chest was crushed—"Don't worry," they said. Just the after-effects of the ventilator and my lungs being turned off for eight hours; and

4. that I was thirsty like I've never been, but the nurse wouldn't let me have water, else I might throw up, faint from the pain, and get pneumonia.... "Here, have some ice chips, but don't swallow the melt...." Great. Crushed ice-chip pebbles, one-at-a-time on my tongue, but Don't Swallow?? Can hardly believe it...can hardly breathe...go feed the meter....

the recovery parade

Watching patients outside my hospital room shuffling round the 14th floor—two, three, five days after major surgery—where they test their legs and upright powers. Being sort of amazed, racked with nonstop aching torso pain, that I'm soon walking beside them, even with mega-doses of morphine and epidural infusions in my spine, even if in Cro-Magnon man fashion, less than 70 hours after waking up, minus one tumor and minus one colon.

catheter blues

Glad, really glad, I wasn't conscious when they shoved the rubber tube through my penis and urethra and into my bladder during surgery. Watching roller-coaster rivulets of pee move out of me every few hours. It stings sometimes; other times I shudder from terrific, searing bladder spasms after I'm done, robbing me of what-ever hint of genital pleasure a "normal" good piss might provide. As my surgeon would say, "Those tissues are angry down there. They don't like what we've done to them." Neither, for the moment, do I.

the endorsement: the bag [part I]

Leaning forward in her chair, Susan Barbour, nurse on the colorectal-surgery floor, patiently explains it all to me: how the colostomy/ileostomy bag works, the hassles and tricks, and even a fashion tip or two for when I rejoin the real world, cancer-free. "So, how do you feel about it?"

Takes a while to answer her, as I guess I have two answers. "I'm thinking about it as if I have a handicap," I say, "but a very small handicap. That's how I feel about it. Basically, I don't want my life controlled by body waste."

a firm future?

No way to prep for it, but two days after they pull my catheter, while peeing into a plastic urinal, I see the beginnings of an erection happening. Beginnings get all the way to middles...which makes me think they were pretty damn successful during surgery and makes me later blurt to Paula across the room: "Don't forget to tell Dr. Welton about my erection this morning."

She tells him while on the phone; I see her smile at his response. He says, "I think this might be the first time I've been so happy about another man's erection. I'll have to tell my wife about this." I'm happy and all, having seemingly dodged Viagra-dependence... but I'm still bedbound, in pain, being fed a couple bags of fluids a day...400 calories each plus ice chips—"No swallowing the melt!"—wondering, well, should he have sounded that surprised?

a "beautiful" stoma

Not one but two or three nurses who've viewed my carved-up body have commented on the craftsmanship of my colorectal surgeon: "A beautiful stoma," one says. "Oh, your stoma looks great," says another. "Really nice."

This does not exactly sink in. For where I used to have a flat lower right abdomen, I now have a ruddy, sturdy, slippery, inch-high plug of intestinal protrusion, a stoma they call it, a beautiful stoma they call it sometimes, a rerouting of small intestine that will serve as an anchor of sorts for the plastic bags I will fasten to my lower torso, which will collect my crap round-the-clock. I am cancer-free, with a good prognosis. And a beautiful stoma.

currency exchange

Phone rings, I pick up. It's Marsha, our friend, who's been there since Day One after diagnosis, who was there in the waiting area the day of surgery, and after....

"Hi, Curt," she says, which tells me she's back from vacation in Costa Rica. "We brought you some extra *colones*," she adds. Turns out the colon—ironically or not—is the unit of currency in Costa Rica. So maybe I should pay my surgeon with 'em?

cheating on my wife

Waiting for Doc Welton to come in the exam room and check his/ my stitches and see how I'm doing post-op, when I spot a scale across the hall....

I strip off my jacket and step on, watching the needle on the dial spin round twice...100 pounds...then 150 and still climbing...to 164. Paula peers over my right shoulder as I shuffle my feet slightly, then some more, and watch the needle creep up to 167. I'm cheating, in full view of my wife. I want her to see me as stronger, bigger, healthier than I was on that horrid day in the hospital seven days post-op when I hardly tipped the scales at 153. Unlike cheating husbands, hospital scales don't lie.

box score

Odds are in, two weeks after surgery, and I'm okay with them:

- ◎ I should have 70 percent of my strength back three months after surgery.

- ◎ I should have 90 percent of my strength after six months (barring complications).

- ◎ I am taking 17 pills a day—eight of them narcotics—to relieve the pain from my operation.

- ◎ There's a better-than-60-percent chance that I'll be colon-cancer-free five years from now.

the endorsement: the bag [part II]

It is not exactly pretty; it is something I am not exactly proud of. The bag I now wear, along with thousands of other colorectal-cancer survivors, is an opaque, white-trimmed polyethylene utensil not that different in shape or appearance from a flattened, up-side-down, old-fashioned milk bottle, the kind you see at carnivals and county fairs–three throws for a dollar...knock 'em off the table...for the big-ass stuffed animal!

The bag is two fists tall or thereabouts, reaching, as I stand, from next to my navel to the glans of my (nonerect) penis. The bag, also called "the pouch" by ostomy experts, is emptied three times a day and at bedtime and changed every three days or so. Featuring two openings—one that attaches to my lower torso with skin-friendly adhesives, the other that empties into the toilet and clips shut—the bag is a lot better alternative than an adult diaper, I'd say; others might say, cynically, "That Depends." I would not however say that. For the bag is airtight-watertight-hygienic. Even as it is not exactly attractive.

"You can wear it under your trunks while swimming," a forthright nurse tells me the other day. This I ponder for more than a minute. For I realize that my swim trunks aren't exactly attractive. Nor, on even my best days at the RallySport Health Club pool, are they something I am exactly proud of. But they do the job. So, it seems, does the bag.

sex and my cancer [part V]

A few weeks after surgery—more than three, but who's counting?— I'm fooling around in bed with Paula, and it feels like high school fooling-around-in-bed.... Because, honestly, I don't know what will happen...on my side of the bed...if we keep this up. Fact is...plumbing's been shut off for a while. Lotsa hands, more than usual, it seems. And I'm not thinking about baseball or the Queen Mother; I'm thinking, for a few seconds at least, about Peter Carroll, M.D., and his finely trimmed mustache and glasses and his ultraclean office and the meeting we had in late March, when he warned me that I might be Viagra-dependent...for a while. For a long while.

Maybe for decades...but...not...now.... "First time since surgery," I'm thinking, feeling a lot like in high school right now, with lotsa hands...and an odd, resurgent, genital-tickle-toward-inevitability... and a rhythmic pumping in the erection that almost wasn't...hold on...on the verge...of bringing unfamiliar groans of pleasure.

Feels so good I feel like shouting but I don't. Instead I'll just write about it, quietly, in the pages of a national magazine. And maybe take a nap.

post-op pep talk

"So," says my best friend, Geoff, settling in for a visit after flying himself and his family halfway across the country to see me soon after surgery, "lemme see the bag."

He's not talking lost luggage from the flight. He means the bag that holds my poo.

"Okay," I say, knowing he'd ask, "but first drop your pants and bend over." He doesn't laugh. Or drop trou.

"You've seen one before," he says.

"Not yours," I say.

He smiles: "I guess they're the same thing, huh?"

Guess so.

surgical strike

Three weeks ago today, a couple of doctors I knew, and eight of whom I didn't, gathered in the OR of Moffitt Hospital to put me under, take me apart, and put me back together. They gathered that Tuesday in April to try to make me a patient who used to have cancer. They gathered to take on a disease that grew for years by division-cell division—and yet the success of their surgery would hinge on collaboration.

There would be no room for error, really. A strike in baseball—"*Steeee-riiike!!!*"—means a pitcher's hit his target A successful surgical strike in cancer-speak means They Got It All, with "clear margins." Turns out the sonsaguns done committed a successful surgical strike, oncologically speaking. Sonsagun surgeons, Dr. Mark Lane Welton and Dr. Peter Carroll, came strutting down the hall after eight hours of tough surgery on my body and my malignancy; sonsaguns came down the hall in their surgical blues, smiling like they'd done roped the biggest mean-ol' steer at the state fair ro-de-o. I'd tip my 10-gallon to 'em, but I'm still unconscious, waiting to wake up in the recovery room and hear Paula repeat what the doctors told me but I did not hear: that I am cancer-free. For now at least; hopefully, till the day I die. Of other causes. Sonsaguns hit the mitt.

Following treatment and surgery, post-op chemotherapy began on schedule.

post-op prognosis [part I]

ESTABLISHING SHOT: Helicopter cam pans south from Golden Gate Bridge and yacht-infested Marina to the cluster of medical buildings crammed into a hill beneath Twin Peaks....

INTERIOR: Sixth-floor exam room, Surgery Faculty Practice Building, University of California, San Francisco, 400 Parnassus Avenue.

"We couldn't have been happier with the way [surgery] went," says Doc Welton, my trusty colorectal surgeon. But when I ask half kiddingly, *"Then why do we need to do chemo?"* he mentions the possibilities of microscopic cells left behind that could mean Big Trouble later.

"We're trying to predict the behavior of a tumor, and we can't do that yet," Doc Welton says. It seems even the most successful surgery can't account for pre-cancerous cells too small to be seen. So then, chemo-time to be safe.

SYNOPSIS: Surgery a success; so too the pre-op radiation and chemo. Still, they're gonna hook me up and infuse me; they're gonna burn the village to save the village.

f-u

Listening intently as Dr. Venook lays it out forthrightly a few days before my first big IV blast. "We use two drugs in combination," he says. One they've already pumped into my body before surgery, 5-fluorouracil (5-FU—or just "F-U" to colon-cancer veterans), and leucovorin, an acid, a cousin to folic acid, that helps the 5-FU do its thing. I'm doing my best to consider this course of chemo "preventive." Just can't wait for side effects like vomiting, nausea, hair loss, weight loss, infection. You know, minor things when compared with "locally invasive" cancer like I had…. Still, I'm not breathing too easily…. "There's a third drug that some centers were experimenting with," Venook adds, "but three deaths were recently reported in clinical trials." We'll stick with the first two drugs then.

[Note: see pg. 118 for updated chemo/biotherapy regimens]

down-and-up

Getting tired of the post-op routine: two hours down, 45 minutes up, waiting for my abdomen muscles, anal stitches, and innards to heal…. Can't sit yet. Comfortably, that is. Couple hours of work, a meal here, a meal there, some TV….

Two weeks out of the hospital and I'm still, basically, horizontal. Or walking, slowly, sorta upright. It's a start.

call it smackey

Waking up one morning in week four of chemo with a small pool of metallic saliva on the back of my tongue. Saliva's telling me my body—my bone marrow actually—has been thoroughly invaded by the 5-FU and is On the Case. Not quite sick enough to throw up; not quite strong enough to shake it off and pretend I'm gonna have a great day. It's a minor part of the assault, unpleasant and tenacious, that attacks my tongue three, four times a week, four, five hours a day, sending copperesque spittle down my gullet; reminding me that I'm still a patient under treatment at an NIH-designated comprehensive cancer center and that more than a few mornings during the rest of my May-June regimen, I will wake up feeling like crap.

The feeling makes me smack my tongue to the roof of my mouth—once, twice, thrice....[My wife] Paula now knows the sound and what it means. Call it smackey, she says. So I do. And suck on a butterscotch, to *beat smackey down.*

the metallic-mouth diet

First thing chemo does some days is mess with the taste buds. There are days when I can't eat fish, chicken, meat, eggs, greens, tomato sauce, or hot *anything* without feeling sick.

Today, like many days, Haagen-Dazs is my dinner.

magic fingers

Watching as our friend and massage therapist, James, walks into the living room lugging his fold-up, fold-out table, getting ready to set up and work on Paula's and my dad's stressed and sore backs.

Knowing full well that I could use, at this point of my recovery, something approximating a friendly, warm touch, but, truth is, I don't want anybody touching me, not now, not for a while; for I have been touched, poked, stuck, burned, inspected, opened, rearranged, closed, and inspected some more by so many strangers and almost-strangers in the last three months that my mind tells my body not to trust anyone not married to me whose fingers and hands want to get close to me. For now, three weeks after surgery, it's all too much. And I recoil: No touching, not yet.

surgeon speak

Today Doc Welton tells me, at four weeks post-op (after I complain about feeling trapped indoors): "That's how you know you're getting better: When you start getting ticked off about not being able to get out and do things, you're healing." Yeah, right.

who is this woman lying next to me?

Because of my surgery, because of my drugs, I cannot write the three paragraphs that follow. I'll need a little help (once again) from my wife, this time from her journal.

Sometimes Curt's memory is foggy. No, actually his memory is sometimes gone. If he acted goofy I might expect it, but he looks me in the eyes, smiles, and agrees to something and then later doesn't recall the conversation ever took place. (Apparently, after you have an eight-hour surgery, anesthesia, chemo, and are taking long-term narcotics for pain, your short-term memory takes a beating.)

It's hard for me to believe that Dr. Welton stood at the foot of Curt's bed telling him, "After seeing your tumor, I'm convinced it was at least eight to 10 years old." Later, I hear Curt telling a friend about his "five-year-old tumor." I tell him what Dr. Welton had said about it being eight to 10 years old, and he looks at me completely shocked and asks, "Did he really say that? When?"

People show up at our door that I'm not expecting and who have called to ask if I need anything because they're on their way. Lately Curt has been forgetting phone calls. Or parts of calls. Out of character. Because of this, I'm afraid for Curt to go to any doctor appointments alone. I'm there to mentally record the conversations, just in case. I am told by Dr. Welton that the forgetfulness is completely normal and shouldn't last more than a year. Curt looks at me every night and tells me he loves me; that I know—but is he really talking to me?

post-op prognosis [part II]

INTERIOR: Darkened bedroom, 5:30 a.m., camera push [wife's POV] into husband rolling slowly out of bed.

CUT TO: Int. bathroom dimly lit, mirror shot reveals husband standing in front of toilet with doughnut-sized ring of pee on Calvin Klein boxers.

Son...of...a...body, don't break down on me now...waking up at dawn to pee, easing my aching body, face up, off the bed into upright position with strategic use of elbow power and knee leverage (I look and feel like a damn Dungeness crab), and flicking on the bathroom light: Something's wrong. There, on my gray cotton underwear, to the right of where my penis resides, is a spot, a wet spot, bigger than a quarter, a lot bigger than a quarter. My eyes lock in on the spot, or rather the reflection of the spot in the bathroom mirror. I don't believe it: After what I've been through, from life-threatening diagnosis through chemo/radiation, bone-racking pain to setbacks and major, life-saving surgery, now I've got to suffer the indignity of a leaking hose?

Not quite 12 hours later, my surgeons have slipped me into their schedules to see what's up, bladderwise. Did they nick a urogenital nerve somewhere during surgery? No time to ponder possibilities I have no clue about; it's time to piss into a "Flowmeter" contraption in the urology clinic, a spinning disc beneath a large funnel, set up atop a toilet that measures urine volume and force of the stream. These are things I've never had checked before, as I'm not a 78-year-old with prostate troubles. But I whip it out, hit the target, and watch a needle record my output.

Then it's flush, wash up, and hop over to the ultrasound room, where Nurse Dora squirts cold jelly on my belly—"Watch the incision stitches," I plead—and starts pressing on me with a wand as she looks for the grainy shadows of my bladder on screen. Seems at first glance I'm "emptying okay"; seems that my stop/start mechanisms of urination are in working order as well. For now, docs think the trouble's not uro-mechanical but actually a side effect: As I'm still healing from the surgery, still popping 17 pain pills round the clock, I'm sleeping "better," longer, more soundly, than I've slept in months. And as the pain eases each week, the narcotics apparently put me under so deeply that I don't feel the first inner twinges of taking a piss that normally would wake me. After all, docs point out, the urine leaking ain't happening during the day when I'm awake (as it does with many prostate-cancer patients)....

Feeling better now about half of my excretionary equipment, feeling that even though my colon and rectum were removed, maybe I won't need bladder surgery to fix my powers of urination. Unfortunately, I'm supposed to make a follow-up appointment. Unfortunately I'll be back.

SYNOPSIS: Seems to me, if life were fair, a recovering cancer patient who craps in a bag shouldn't have to worry about a leaky dick.

sex and my cancer [part VI]

Stumbling upon the startling statement in a "Chemotherapy and You" brochure: "It is advisable to wear a condom during intercourse for up to 48 hours after treatment, as chemotherapy drugs may be present in sperm," and at once being taken aback and frightened. For me and for Paula, who I may be unwittingly poisoning. "Nobody told me this," I'm thinking, while hurriedly doing the math. I breathe easier when it computes: It's been at least 72 hours since my last dose of chemo. So last night was okay. In more ways than one.

dr. worthless...
still completely worthless

Phone rings. Paula answers. It's Dr. Fuller, her OB-GYN, calling from Denver to see how we're doing...it reminds me that he's called four times since my diagnosis, and my ex-gastro, Dr. Worthless, who missed what they now think was an eight-to-ten-year-old rectal tumor three and a half years ago during a screening colonoscopy, hasn't called since December. Reminds me also of the two visits I made to Worthless last summer and fall, complaining of rectal pain each time but not receiving a basic, digital rectal exam either time.

All this sends me to the Net, to a leading malpractice lawyer's Website and then further...where I soon learn Dr. Worthless's Colorado medical board "license status" is "active" and also learn that there is "no disciplinary information on file."

Not yet, anyway.

pot luck

In my left hand, I hold a plastic card that has my picture on it, a card issued by the San Francisco Department of Public Health. It reads: "Medical Cannabis Voluntary Identification Program. Issue Date: 29-Mar-01; Expires: 29-Mar-02." I use this card when making legal purchases. In my right hand, I hold a newspaper clipping, front-page story, of the *San Francisco Chronicle* that reads: MEDICINAL POT RULED ILLEGAL

In my recent memory, I hold an image of me, lying on our couch, moaning in severe pain, arms at my side, fists clenched, kicking my legs in staccato spasms, trying to send the pain from a Stage-3 tumor lodged in my pelvis out of my body and out of my mind.

In my not-so-recent memory, I hold an image of me driving a car, cocking my head in disbelief at a proposed Supreme Court Justice, Clarence Thomas, in a Senate hearing in D.C, being accused by a college law professor, Anita Hill, of sexually harassing her in part by telling her he found a pubic hair atop a can of Coca-Cola that was on his desk. I wondered then, What could he possibly have been thinking?

In my left hand, I hold a recent weekly newspaper clipping from a wire service that says Clarence Thomas found that "medical necessity is not a defense to manufacturing and distributing marijuana." I wonder now, halfway through chemo, What could he possibly be thinking?

derailed

"Once you've been hit by the train so many times," Paula tells me in bed this morning, "you're afraid to stand on the tracks to see if another one's coming." No wonder my wonderful wife is scared at this point in my treatment...it's time to schedule the first series of "follow-up" CT scans. We know the drill: head, chest, abdomen, pelvis. Send some ultra-energy X-ray beams through my organs and bones and see what shows up on film....

"...so many times..." Paula saying about the train makes me think: I've been hit once—and good—by the Colorectal Express... whereas she recalls, and for good reason, five derailments:

◎ 1994, her niece, our niece, Sandra, getting hit by a logging truck on a Sierra mountain road, falling into a coma for 14 months, and still recovering from brain damage seven years later....

◎ 1994, her brother, Larry, falling 30 feet off a roof on a house he was painting, landing facedown and surviving, being medevacked and plastic-surgically put back together, one facial bone at a time....

◎ 1997, suffering a life-threatening ruptured ectopic pregnancy that sent her tumbling to the floor and into surgery while her blood pressure read an absolutely mind-numbing 50/0. (I didn't even know you could have zero BP and survive....)

◎ 1999, while out of town on a job, finding a lump in her throat, lodged deeply in her thyroid, causing docs to operate and me to forever associate driving across the Golden Gate Bridge, alone, into San Francisco, with heading to the hospital to get her post-op results from pathology. TGIB, Thank God It's Benign, we were able to say....

And, hey, not to worry for a while...till December 2000, when that last frickin' choo-choo decided to derail me, her, both of us, I guess, which is why I might be a little more scared of those upcoming CTs, come to think of it, than I'm letting on. Even though they come back negative for cancer, I'll always need to be prepared for The Next Scan.

halfway home?

Flipping the page on the calendar, saying so long to May, seeing how many days we have left in San Francisco—for treatment and packing—and focusing on June 17. Then it's home to Denver/ Boulder for final chemo and settling back in.

Got the diagnosis in late December; started treatment in early January. Got six weeks of radiation/chemo in January and February, rad burns finally healed in late March.

Got operated on in early April in a major way; finally healed in— what am I talking about, it's early June and I still haven't "finally" healed. Can't even roll all the way over in bed, for the cut stomach muscles that still ache daily and deeply.

Got six weeks of chemo in May and June; have six more to go before I flip the calendar past July and August. Somehow, by my count, feels like I am only halfway home. Go figure.

chemo-by-the-bay

Easing into a leatherette La-Z-Boy in the UCSF infusion center, waiting for my blood work and for two friends to come by. (Farley's a San Fran local; Pete'll fly in from Denver for a few hours.) Suddenly I hear Paula say, "Oh, my God, there's Brandy!"—meaning my grade-school friend who's joined by my high-school bud Jerry, which means we're having a surprise San Francisco-chemo-by-the-Bay party, only half of which I was expecting....

Can't believe these guys pulled this one off—that with four wives and 13 kids among them, they were able to shuck their schedules, blow off clients, and see if they couldn't give me some old-style, are-we-ever-gonna-grow-up, ball-busting support. On a day I might not feel much like partying.

For the occasion, Farley rents a 1450cc Harley (which Brandy falls off of while stopped at a stoplight); Pete raids the free (!) graham-crackers-and-apple-juice "for patients only" pantry; and Jerry makes gross jokes about the rubber gloves he doesn't seem to want to take off.... I'm back in high school again, laughing my ass off with old friends...till the drugs make me weak and the airport calls the boys home.

untied

There are days, many days after surgery, that I don't tie my shoes because it hurts too much to bend over. So I tuck the laces under the tongue, making my cross-trainers into loafers, and spare myself the indignity of asking my wife to help me make a bow.

262,800 minutes

Packing up, in our friends Monica's and Chris's home, packing up to go home. Half a year we've lived out of town, or 262,800 minutes if you go by the lyrics of *Rent*, which we saw at the Orpheum the other night. "How do you measure, measure a year?"

Six months of diagnoses and treatment and recoveries and there are still six weeks of chemo sessions left, which I'll get in Denver, under the guidance of my San Fran doctors. Call it aftercare, even if it isn't quite. And if anything should go wrong, really or terribly wrong, I'll be back in San Francisco quick as United Air can take me, for there's a trust I'm not yet willing to share. All these minutes later.

214,600 dollars

Filing the bills that have found us at home, sent from all of the parties who have played a part in my cancer assault. Wondering if and when we're gonna hit the $300,000 mark in assessed billings.

breast cancer and my cancer

Can't stop 'em, but good friends and colleagues are talking to me more about cancer these days, breast cancer and colon cancer mostly, diseases that seem to bring extraordinary surprise to others when they learn of diagnoses that have hit people close to them.

"You're not supposed to get breast cancer at 44," or 38, or whatever, I hear. Same goes for colon cancer or rectal cancer. There's some bond there; as a friend of mine put it, "It's the f---ed-upness of a young person getting cancer." Then there's the follow-up f'd-upness of radiation or chemo or both and maybe some kind of mental bluesy funk when all the bad cells have been exterminated.

There's something else, too: the fact that I worked for seven years for the women's magazine that started the Pink Ribbon Breast Cancer Awareness Campaign. I'm an unlikely cancer vet. I used to write about breast cancer without feeling truly close to it. I can now relate to cancer patients in ways that I couldn't before... whether I like it or not. It's different to talk about it and to write about it...than to have it.

tough day, dude

Strolling out of chemo, glad to have another blast out of the way, walking up to the car, and staring, blankly, at the windshield. Great. Guy goes into the esteemed Rocky Mountain Cancer Center to try to kick cancer's ass; meantime some fake-cop parking jockey sees I've been in there for more than two hours, slaps us with a 15-buck ticket.

Didn't we see *the sign?*

Tough day, dude.

a worse person?

I used to be a happy guy. People say I've always been happy. Haven't felt that way in a while and instead feel that I'm not as nice a person as I used to be. Question is, why am I now less tolerant of other people? Especially after getting tons of support from my family, friends, and incredibly kind strangers. "It's not just getting cancer," Paula says. "It's the threat of getting cancer, facing death, your mortality, that's made you different. You don't have patience for insincerity anymore. Once your security and happiness are threatened, you can't be the same." But am I worse?

unforgiven

While pondering a suit in Denver against my former gastroenterologist, I'm not thinking big $ at all. Hell, I now know (but didn't know three months ago) there's a $1 million medical-malpractice cap in Colorado.

And I know he didn't give me cancer. But the way I see it, the doctor I'm thinking of suing did not practice good medicine upon me. Not even "acceptable" medicine upon me.

He scoped me in '97, missed some advanced rectal cancer (according to another doctor whom I do respect); then failed to perform a digital rectal exam twice when I went to him complaining of rectal pain. When I got my rectal-cancer diagnosis from him in December, I was stunned. Then I got angry. Six months later, whether or not I end up going forward with a lawsuit, he's still unforgiven.

hate letters

Never heard the phrase spoken to me till I got cancer and then got rid of it. Never heard a doctor say, "I get at least a couple of hate letters every year," especially a doctor of mine [Dr. Alan Venook, my oncologist] who's committed to serving patients who now have or have had cancer. Sticks in my mind: "...a couple of hate letters every year." For telling people news they didn't, or don't, want to hear; for telling people they have cancer, and for sometimes telling people they have cancer and that they don't have that many options to fight it. Which means there's a lot of pain going round these halls. And a few painful letters in answer to a new kind of pain. Hate letters, the doctor says. I decide to send the guy a nice note.

insomniac addict

Padding about the bedroom and kitchen in moccasin-slippered feet, in search of Cheerios and milk, wondering what this buzz in my veins could possibly mean, this unfocused energy that's been keeping me up till 3:00 a.m. for days now, or for nights, rather, as my pain subsides and my trip through chemoland begins to feel commonplace.

Thinking to myself (who else would be up at this hour?) that maybe I've been taking too many narcotics lately.

Figuring out, when I wake all groggy and disheveled, fogged-in and angry-tired at 9:00 a.m., feeling like I've been partying or drinking the night before...figuring out that because I've been taking the narcotic Vicodin for pain for five and a half months now and cut the dose by 90 percent over the past 10 days, I'm somehow going through a skittish-sleepless withdrawal.

I've taken Vikes at bedtime since December for cancer and surgery pain—and check with Dr. Mark Welton [my surgeon] the next day about my theory. He doesn't seem worried at all when he says, "Technically, you're addicted. But that doesn't mean you'll be an addict."

I've got to taper down more slowly, he says, and might even still take a Vike at night for a while, until I begin to heal more to the point where I can move around without pain and can physically tire myself out...and so to sleep.

But not at this moment, in the dark hours between 2:00 and 4:00 a.m. on a Monday that's not starting out well. I'm hooked, for the time being. I'm an up-all-night, cancer-free, recovering colon-cancer patient who now has another health problem with which to concern himself.

chemo-by-the-rockies

Chemo blows. It's "toxic medicine" to some, wickedly effective for others. It's methodically pumped into my veins by a Sigma infusion pump that has a "syringe holder" feature and an "air upstream occlusion" alarm. The chemo finds its way into the bone marrow, and that's why its kick is so powerful.

I have the flu. But not quite. I've started another chemotherapy session (my third six-week course), and I am nauseated for at least a few hours, sometimes up to eight or 10 hours a day. But I don't have the flu, not quite, and I don't throw up. If I were a guy who paid no mind to post-feminist culture, I'd liken my nausea to that suffered in the early terms of pregnancy...except...here I am taking electro-pumped poison to kill some potentially malignant cells that would kill me if I didn't try to fight them. But I'm fighting what I can't feel and what the doctors can't see or guarantee is still there—microscopic pre-cancerous cells in my body. The stuff may work; in reality it does quite often. Nonetheless, chemo blows.

weed...be...gone

Bending down in the backyard, still moving in slow-mo post-surgical fashion, to grab hold of a dandelion-gone-beanstalk in the raised garden bed, to take back some of the earth that's gone wild with weedy growths since we've been off fighting some cancer in San Francisco....

Ripping out some grass as I yank the weed in my gloved right hand, taking out more dirt than I intend to, flashing back to the talk I had with Doc Welton after my surgery: "What does it feel like to take out tumor?" I ask, invoking some faux O.R.-speak. "You cut—and then pull," he answers. "You cut tension. It's like pulling sod up from the ground...you pull a 'corner' till it's taut, then cut, then pull some more, and cut away at the point of tension."

Okay, then, when you're a colorectal surgeon like Welton, you don't take tumor timidly. "In my residency," he tells me later, "I had one chief [resident] who told me, when you're operating on a cancer patient and he's open from above, you don't stop cutting till you see the table." Don't know why the good doc shared that one with me—on second thought, I'd asked him. And the tension part hits home. I grab the next Mr. Evil Weed, dig my fingers down, and pull down below ground line. I pull like someone who's decidedly not feeling sorry for wayward greenery today. I get it out, root and all, and toss it in the pile that'll end up in the 30-gallon Cinch Sak Hefty Bag...no need to send that sucker to pathology.

a dozen words about death

Oddly, I feel no closer to death than I did last December.

3:47 a.m.

Waking up wired, after going to bed wired, "addicted" or "Vicodin-dependent"—who gives a shit what it's called—any which way, it feels like two dozen bees are buzzing in my chest, shoulders, and arms...and suddenly I have empathy for Matthew Frickin' Perry, for chrissakes. Doc Welton says it could take weeks to kick; Doc Venook concurs. Doc Cohn [Dr. Allen Cohn, my new oncologist in Denver] talks up Benadryl a bit. Paula wants to feed my face nocturnally to get me through this withdrawal.

This is great: Try OTC antihistamines; feed the bees. But all I want is some z's.

post-op prognosis [part III]

INTERIOR: Harshly lit windowless exam room #10, Rocky Mountain Cancer Center, Denver. Paula's POV of Dr. Allen Cohn palpating my torso with his fingers.

CUT TO: Closeup of Dr. Cohn's face, looking unconcerned, as his circling index and middle fingers stop on my chest, upper right quadrant.

"This mole needs to come off," he says.

CUT TO: My face looking seemingly unconcerned.

"I've had that checked before," I say.

CUT TO: Paula's face, looking concerned.

CUT TO: 3-Shot, push-in to Dr. Cohn.

"I'd feel better if it were in a jar," Dr. Cohn says.

SYNOPSIS: In less than three weeks, it will be. I'm going to have a new dermatologist. It's never too soon to prevent cancer.

the celebrity of cancer

"They say that people who go through stuff like you've been through," an ex-colleague writes, "have a profoundly changed perspective on life—that surviving something like this can paradoxically make you a happier person than you were before. Any truth to this?"

Hell if I know.

I didn't ask to be Cancer Boy.... I certainly didn't audition. But I have been feeling increasingly weird over the past six months, not just physically but about how people treat me, at times making me seem like a B-list celebrity.

It's almost freakish. That because of my biology—and the anti-cancer assault that was thrown at it—people act like in some way I might be closer to God. I've been into the fire—and come back. Maybe they think I've gone into the fire for them, or, rather, instead of them. Some people say I'm brave, but let's be frank here, I didn't walk into the fire willingly. I am not exalted. Any time you do something out of the ordinary, people want to get closer to you. Thing is, this comes at a time when I typically feel like crap a few hours a day, and all I want sometimes is distance— from just about everybody.

getting my life back

Kicked my cup-a-day coffee habit through the first two rounds of chemo and didn't seem to miss it. But I've started up again at home, maybe trying to make things the same as before....

Unfroze the health-club membership in July, even though my weight lifting's restricted, trying to make me as strong as before....

Got used to waking up same time as Paula every day for months, when I needed her caregiving more; now I wake up earlier most days, same as before....Got our dog, Bolder, back the other day, chauffeured in from Chicago in the backseat of my folks' car, trying to make things nearly the same as before....It's one thing to have your life handed back to you by your doctors; it's quite another to get that life back same as before.

a better person?

Dropping down out of the clouds, touching down on a sunbaked runway near our Colorado home, I am happy/sad/half-healed/scared. For now, I am 912 (air) miles away from the doctors who saved my life. I am grateful. I am healthy, after 20-some weeks of cancer treatment and extraordinarily successful surgery. I am, again, in a position where I can say I have my life ahead of me. But am I a better person?

I've read Joyce Wadler's book, *My Breast*, in which she emerges on the back side of her cancer treatment a better woman than when she first got her gloomy biopsy results in New York City. I've read Lance Armstrong's best-seller, *It's Not About the Bike*, about his testicular cancer, recovery, and post-op Tour de France glory. Amazingly, he writes that knowing what he knows now, if he had to choose between having cancer and winning the Tour de France, he'd choose cancer. He's now a better guy. I've heard Eric Davis of the San Francisco Giants on the radio, talking about his bout with colon cancer and how it's so curable when caught early. He may be a better person, but let's be honest: He's hitting all of .198 heading into August. So many cancer-recovery stories end with an upbeat notion. That's understandable. That's admirable even. But too many of these stories end with the notion that somehow, through all the pain, their cancer has made them "a better person." This one won't.

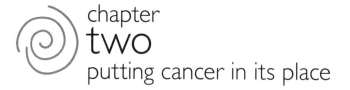

chapter
two
putting cancer in its place

There's no easy way to say it, because cancer isn't easy: After all that's been thrown at us, one of the toughest challenges for any cancer patient is to move on, to trade in our medical status, to stop being a patient and start being a former patient. No matter what the pathology reports say about "clear margins" (or not exactly clear), the idea of cancer in our bodies Does Not Leave. Sure, there may be no more daily doc visits or phone calls. No weekly "bloods." No more sessions hooked up to the auto-chemo pump-on-wheels. All good. But by extension there's also a tremendous loss of support once treatment has wound down. What do you do? Now that you're *normal* again? You wait a few years, hopefully, then a couple more. You do this until maybe the 5-year mark, when you're officially, medically "cured." This is a long flippin' time.

At the same time this transition is surely not as physically tough as radiation or chemotherapy. And it's not nearly as nerve-searing painful as what you felt when your tumor was first treated. Still, there's no easy way to say it because there's no easy way to do it: How do you shrink the heavy, mindful space that cancer has introduced in your day-to-day thinking, for weeks or months at a time? The fear was—and is—so real. Mortality made itself known, ahead of schedule, in your life, in your house. (Survivors know this stat too well: about 50,000 people die of colorectal cancer in the U.S. each year, or enough to fill the seats of New York's Yankee Stadium).

So when it comes to handling these haunting fears, it turns out there's a huge difference between putting cancer behind you and putting cancer "in its place." For countless numbers of my fellow survivors agree: We will never completely put it behind us. It's part of who we are as long as we live. We can, however, with some time and help, put it in a reasonable, psychological space. (I'll not soon forget the oncology nurse at UCSF who once told me, maybe a month too soon, "You're gonna' have to deal with the Bogey Man in the closet for the rest of your life," she said. "The trick is to figure out how wide you're gonna decide to leave the door open each day.") Um, okay.... The rest of this chapter looks at how patients like me, and you, and caregivers, actually do that. It's a psychological bind patients don't often talk about, at least not often enough. They see managing their cancer emotions, as I did after a nine-month treatment and surgery protocol a few years ago, as another burden. If you acknowledge you "still" have daily, weekly, whatever thoughts about recurrence, you're being honest, yes. But at the same time you're then succumbing to certain fears. And nobody wants to think about themselves as weak at a time when they are expected, rather suddenly and by so many others, to Be Strong.

Unlike the key two-year mark that colon cancer patients first set in their sights (because "of all the people who have recurrences, 80 percent of those will develop within the first two years," says Allen Cohn, M.D., of Rocky Mountain Cancer Centers in Denver), the precise time at which patient becomes ex-patient isn't in any of the medical books. It's amorphous: could be one month, or 2.5 years; and it could be never. It's tricky for patients or loved ones to wrap their arms around, even in the most treatable cases. And for most that relatively peaceful feeling doesn't arrive quickly enough.

re-intro, re-entry

In my case, the time after post-op was a bit jittery. As I wrote in my journal after I'd left the hospital worlds: "Two years since diagnosis, and I am cancer free. Don't call myself a survivor...yet; feels too early. Don't call myself a 'warrior,' either. That's for the charity-fund appeal and pink-ribbon ad-campaign writers. But I've taken nine months of radiation ('We're gonna pound you,' my radiation doc said.); recovered from life-saving surgery with most of my body intact; adopted a child; and I have started hugging my family and friends a bit harder.

Call me middle-aged guy in remission—make that recovery—because the way I see it, remission means merely temporary absence of disease. Call me healthy but wary. Been bouncing back and forth from the U.S. to London, where Paula is once again working as associate producer on the *Harry Potter* films. Been writing again, even some new kinds of stuff for a TV documentary I'm trying to get made. Been getting used to getting cancer behind me, even if it'll always seem ahead of me. Also been getting used to being a new dad, to giving all sorts of care at all hours to Baby Josh, kind-of-like Paula did for me. Still don't feel, though, that beating advanced colon cancer has made me a 'better man.' Even if I am, I've noticed, more apt to sign off letters, cards and notes with 'love.' "

Paula, by contrast, didn't see me as "healthy but wary" at this juncture. I looked in her journal (with her permission, I swear) and found she's already sort-of-told me how I was putting cancer in its place:

"he's livin'"

"Back in England, I find I'm living with a forty-four-year old teenager. Curt won't be where he doesn't want to be, or with whom he doesn't want to be with. He's spontaneous and seizing the moment, not wasting time with small talk, pretending he's interested. He went

to a play on a whim on Friday...'Rent' (again)...with some college kids he didn't know who had an extra cheap ticket to spare. He ran into them in Leicester Square. I tell him I was worried. Couldn't reach him for hours. "I'm livin'! he said, and thank God he is."

three times a year

Less than three months later Paula told how *she's* putting cancer in its place. Or trying to....

"I'm in a lot better place now, I guess because it's January. Next scans aren't till the end of April. That's because Dr. Cohn says, 'CTs every three to four months (for the first two years after surgery; then every six months).' And Curt's figured out, if we stretch it out till four, that's one less per year, plus less radiation from the scans.

"I find myself now living my life with this benchmark. So far relieved, and filled with joy, but as the weeks pass, feeling the dread that slowly creeps up on me, as the next trip home gets closer. When we sit in the oncologist's office, trying to anticipate and read into his every expression...hearts-are-racing...then learning he hasn't read them yet; he'll be right back....Trying to hear the pace of his footsteps as he returns to see if they will give me any insight as to the news about to be delivered: Do we get to continue our lives as they are—so full of love and joy, and our new baby, Joshua...or do we put on our gear again and go into to the fire and fight for life?"

"i don't wanna talk about it"

In the mid-1990s, Judy Webster, 57, of Omaha, Nebraska, survived a diagnosis of advanced colon cancer. It was only after she'd had emergency surgery and mostly healed that she realized people of all stripes—even family members—weren't at all comfortable talking about...the certain kind of cancer that she'd had. The one that attached to her bowels.

"In 1996, people didn't talk about colon cancer," Webster says. "When I left the hospital I felt very alone. No one reached out to me, like they do for breast cancer patients [today]. The nurses were very kind, but when I went home...that was it. I just felt really alone; my cancer was not talked about. If you [walked and] went around somebody, they would just stare at you." Imagine, trying to re-enter a family situation, as it was, and being stared at, because of the *kind* of cancer you've suffered. "I do have a handful of friends that were more open. But friends, my husband's co-workers, they were afraid to say anything to me. Nowadays, there's a better understanding of it. There's openness; more education. And more understanding by the general public. So now they'll know, and maybe be able to say, 'Hey, you have colon cancer, that doesn't mean you're going to die.' When I got out of the hospital, it was like breast cancer was [considered] 30 years ago—just was not talked about at all...now it's okay to talk about it."

Not only is it 'okay' to talk about today, it turns out this kind of talk may even hold some partly-understood, powerful health and longevity benefits. According to David Spiegel, M.D., of Stanford University Medical Center in Palo Alto, California, who has studied cancer patients and talk therapy for more than 15 years, certain research trials have shown that cancer and ex-cancer patients who join support groups and "download" stresses and fears (also, joys) in group settings tend to fair better, survival-wise, than similar patients who have tended to go it alone. An important note, however, needs to be mentioned: As perhaps exciting as Dr. Spiegel's and colleagues' work has appeared, this is an *observed* relation between longevity and group therapy. It has not been proven that talk therapy is *responsible* for the increases in longevity that have been reported.

"Helping people handle the stress of cancer can help patients live longer," claims Dr. Spiegel, a world-renowned clinician. "Such help includes expressive group therapy, building bonds with other [patients] in the same situation, expressing their emotions, detoxifying dying, using self-hypnosis for pain, and reordering their priorities in life."

how different are you now?

Although I had only been to a handful of cancer support group sessions when I started writing this book, I felt, at times, that writing about my case in a national magazine a few years earlier gave me some of the advantages of being in a group. It became, over time, therapeutic for me to "vent" on paper and onscreen. When I started writing about how cancer felt, however, I didn't know why I did it. As a writer it simply felt normal. (In a similar, more visually artistic vein, the British photographer and videographer, Sam Taylor-Wood, made a quite remarkable picture two years after her colon cancer treatment and immediately after her treatment for breast cancer. It is entitled: "Self Portrait as a Tree," and is as beautiful as it is haunting.) In addition, through writing about my case I felt some of the support-group "lift" without having made an actual link with a Colorado-based group my first year home. All the while, friends and others kept peppering me with questions about healing that helped me maybe more than I knew at the time. Such as:

"Are you doing okay? And, "What do you think caused it?"

"I don't know," I've said, in answer to both questions, at different times. What I know is I've now lived years with cancer (without even knowing it), and a few years with a body that can be called "cancer-free." I don't believe I am "happier" than I was five years ago. But I'm beginning to put cancer in its place; for now, that means not quite behind me. Which seems normal, at least to me.

not exactly normal

"My life will never be whatever normal is," said Lisa Dubow, 47, of Los Angeles, a Stage 4 patient who surprised–time and again– teams of researchers with her resilience and healing abilities since her diagnosis and first treatments in 2001. "It wasn't normal before, but this gives me more passion to become active, to give me more time to be more politically active, and the joy of seeing a change in my life." When Dubow talked about political activism, for her that meant health activism more so than traditional Democrat/ Republican U.S. politics. Specifically, she served as a state coordinator for the Colon Cancer Alliance and as a board member of Fight Colorectal Cancer.

"And to be honest," Dubow said, "I've actually guided people [toward research trials, new drugs]. I'm not a doctor, but I've guided people to certain doctors; I have saved certain people's lives, and it's awesome."

[Editor's note: Advocate Lisa Dubow passed away in July, 2007. A fund in her honor that spurs research to fight late-stage cancer, is at http://fightcolorectalcancer.org/research/lisa-fund.]

The more I've talked with patients and their families, the more I've found we aren't all afraid to shed our formerly protective habits. This is a tough transition for some; a bit less so for others.... Talking about colon cancer surely wasn't easy, at first, for someone like Katie Couric, of NBC's *Today* show, who has mobilized millions of dollars—and people—in support of colon cancer awareness since her late husband, Jay Monahan, died at age 42 of the disease in 1998. Couric even went so far as to broadcast her own colonoscopy on morning television in 2000, as part of Colorectal Cancer Awareness Month. (In fact, a few years later she told a press conference audience that her colonoscopy on-air "experiment" had to be approved by NBC-TV honcho Jeff Zucker, who not only ran the entertainment network, but was already a colon cancer survivor who had been diagnosed at age 31.)

For the rest of us, especially perhaps men, talking about blood in our stools doesn't come so easily. That may be one reason why men are especially at risk...not a biological disadvantage as much as a cultural one: Middle-aged women, at least, have had decades of experience in talking with doctors about blood, menstrual blood, and how hormones and other bodily changes have affected their menses. This is New Stuff for the male of the species, even if and when we're led to the exam table by a smiling Couric and/or the other women who affect our lives and our health.

survivors' guilt

Then, too, there is still more we (of both genders) don't talk about: After a war, a holocaust, a plane crash, you often hear people talk about "survivors' guilt." It's a known, studied phenomenon in psychology and psychiatry. Some years ago, I interviewed a Denver sales executive who quietly (for a sales guy, that is) had made a few million dollars in telemarketing and consulting. But instead of hanging all manner of corporate plaques hailing his accomplishments on his office walls, he had hung prominently, alongside his desk, a fading newspaper article that reported on a major, 1991 airplane crash in which 180 people had perished in the Midwest. This man, a thyroid cancer survivor, was supposed to be on that plane. He arrived so early, however, that he had qualified for a standby seat on a flight that left just one hour earlier.... Survivor's Guilt, perhaps? After all these years? Or does he continue to hang the harrowing clipping as simply a memento to being in the right place at the right time? He likes to think of this event, this near-death experience, as having more than a little to do with faith. The same goes for countless other cancer patients, I've found since my Stage 3 diagnosis a few years ago.

Sometimes, whether we are ready or not, we're forced to "honor" the threats that have so impacted our lives. And ask the larger questions, the *largest* questions about life.

Having acknowledged this, though, the reason I still don't talk much about this possible guilt is that I still feel too damn hungry to survive. And from where I sit, despite mine and all the "NED" (No evidence of disease) anniversaries of my cancer brethren, I still believe I'm on shaky ground. I feel true empathy for my fellow cancer patients past and present, but the guilt, from a personal standpoint, I can't yet fathom. Perhaps it's because I'm unfeeling (despite appearances or what people who know me well have told me), but I don't honestly think that's the reason I'm not feeling the guilt pangs. Most things considered, the aversion to "celebrating" my survival-to-date probably has to do with a lingering sense of fear instead of finality. Plus, it has to do with a will to not carry others' burdens in ways I know I have in the past. Could it be possible, I wonder, that I won't be totally healed until I feel, acknowledge, even honor the haunting, hangdog emotion of survivor's guilt? If so, it's a stage that will bring up others' states of suffering. It's a stage, then, that I won't especially look forward to "achieving."

survivors' grit

For other patients, who've survived their first scare and yet still harbor cancer cells in their bodies, the up-down day-to-day existence is decidedly more trying than mine has been. For them and still others, it doesn't make emotional or physical sense to try to pretend the cancer's not there. (They don't have the "luxury" to ponder survivors' guilt, at least not yet.)

"I've had so much treatment and have been through two clinical trials," said Dubow "that the research [teams] kind of don't want me any more." With advanced disease, but as someone who outlived a handful of prognoses already, Lisa knew her long-term survival might be tied to continuing to think of herself as a patient…to keep searching for new therapies, new tacks to take when the standard ones played out. She was so steeped in colon cancer medicine fact she knew drug companies didn't necessarily want her on their drug-testing rosters. The reason is: As long as one keeps outliving the expected odds, the researchers following a case might wonder whether it's their particular drug that's responsible…for one's surprising longevity. "To have someone like me [survive] raises the question," Lisa said, matter-of-factly. "Is it their drugs that are working on me, or is it a combination of everything I've had *plus* their drugs? Those are some of the issues I've had."

Or, alternately, as Judy Webster, of Nebraska, says, "I know that life is so precious now, and that I've got to make every moment count…. I was told by my sister, 'Take one day at a time,' and I really think that we all should live that way. People say it…but what does that really mean? That you do have to stop, [slow down]? I'll look at the tree, and nature, and I'll see it in a different way, now. Appreciate it more. And I'll think about people who have died, and I'll think: 'I am here to enjoy these things, I'm going to enjoy them. Maybe this comes from being an artist, when I look at the sky, every night, I think about it. When I see the sunrise, I think about it….

"I think it helps to talk about it," Judy adds, of the survivor's legacy. "And it has gotten better, people in general, I mean. They don't know what to say and they don't want to hurt your feelings. I didn't want to hurt my friends. Actually, what I wanted to do [when I found out about my cancer] was, I wanted to just go over there and hug my friend and hold her, and I couldn't do that either. Because it makes people feel funny. So you have to be 'up,' you have to have hope. And be strong for them because they don't want to see you weak."

"But," she concludes, " don't ever say, 'Oh, I know exactly how you feel.' I don't do that. I just say, 'I can relate to, somewhat, how you feel.' I don't [truly] know how you feel, but I can relate to it."

And Judy could probably relate quite well to what I felt, personally, a couple years ago, when I was still unsure of whether I'd make my two-year-all-clear; still trying to be "up" when so much uncertainty still hung, greasily, in the air....

false alarm?

"Waking on a cold morning, early winter," I wrote, "with a twinge astride my right testicle that ranges from groin to lower torso... uh-oh. Feels a little like a groin pull, but higher and connected to the dull, lingering pains I feel in my lower abdomen when I do push-ups or other ab work (not that I do a lot of 'ab-work.'). Surgery scar tissue, maybe, or worse? I make a note to ask about this pain at the next CT-scan checkup in two months....."

The months passed quickly, but not quickly enough.... "Driving south on Highway 36, heading out of the Boulder foothills and down to Denver," I added, "to see my oncologist, my reader of CT scans of abdomen, of pelvis, of chest, who checks for signs of angry, rogue cells. Passed the one-year mark okay, then the year-and-a-half...but for some reason the year and nine months has me jittery. Maybe it's because I'm a father now, maybe it's because I had that twinge...(though countless ex-cancer patients, I later learn, are forever mistaking twinges for recurrence).

"Here we go...and turns out I have no reason to worry. NED: No evidence of disease. No changes, apparently, from the study four months prior (love the way they call it a "study"). Dr. Cohn walks into the exam room and starts chatting with me about my recent stint in England. 'You likin' it over there?' Good news. If I had cancer signs, he wouldn't be talking tourism. 'You're healthy,' he says. I ask him to repeat this into my Sony micro cassette that

I have placed on the chair next to me...(in case of bad news and my note-taking/thinking/reasoning collapsing). 'He's healthy!' Dr. Cohn says loudly to the Sony and thus to Paula, who will hear this tape at home after the baby wakes up. I smile as if I knew all along all would be okay (as if), and hop out to the car to call home. (You don't shout good news like this into a cell phone inside the Rocky Mountain Cancer Center.... Too many ill patients in attendance.)

"Now I'm back on the road, rolling north toward Highway 36 and home, feeling like I have just graduated from something big, singing along to a Springsteen CD, pounding the steering wheel as a snare drum, or cymbal, as if I'm Tony Soprano in his Escalade.

These are better days, bay-buh |
These are better days it's true |
These are better days, bay-buh |
There's better days shining through.

soldiering on

Besides "Dr." Bruce Springsteen, one Canadian couple I talked with, two years after their Big Scare, helped me see quite clearly that there are better days ahead. They also nearly made me cry, when they talked about trying to put colon cancer behind them, maybe because I saw so much of Paula and myself mirrored back to me. Especially when Jayne, 38, talked about the new baby in the house, born just three months before Kenny's diagnosis in a Toronto hospital a few years ago. Jayne and Kenny, 41, and baby Amy, are out of the woods, you might say. But it wouldn't be quite right to call them gleeful. Least not yet....

"Sometimes I feel embarrassed by my 'notoriety," Jayne says. *"You know, good wishes from long-unseen relatives and the like; you know you're being talked about and that it all sounds 'tragic.' And some-times I feel amiss wondering what friends have noticed about me*

putting fatigue in its place

When your family and friends are calling (you know from Caller ID), it's tough, at first, to ignore the ring, to not answer the phone. But when you're recovering from colorectal cancer—or the chemo or radiation or surgery that's still fighting it—there are times where you know you've got to store your energy for just an hour or two of activity a day. And, cancer patients know too well, talking on the phone (about your body and disease) constitutes activity. Fatigue, we know, is no small matter.

Not long ago, medical researchers found that cancer-related fatigue is more important than they had previously believed. In studies at Moffitt Cancer Center, Tampa, Florida, Dr. Paul Jacobsen and colleagues tried treating fatigue with new substances (i.e., EPO, for anemia-like conditions) and medicines, instead of merely relying on talk therapy…and the passage of time. They were pleasantly, and repeatedly surprised.

"Fatigue is exacerbated by depression, emotional distress and stress," says Dr. Jacobsen. "And cancer patients experience high levels of stress and distress, especially during treatment." Which only, he adds, exacerbates their fatigue. Patients won't always mention their fatigue because they expect it, or feel they should just accept it—the "cancer" part of healing seems more important to discuss.

"It's the silent symptom," Jacobsen adds, "because patients don't realize they are suffering a symptom." Until now, and possibly for months past the last treatment, patients and caregivers haven't realized how many ways there are available to fight fatigue, and to help put this side-effect behind them.

For more info on the studies, or related treatment, contact:
National Colorectal Cancer Research Alliance/ EIF:
1-800-872-3000;
www.nccra.org; or Moffitt Cancer Center, Paul B. Jacobsen, Ph.D.,
813-745-3862.

over the last couple of years. I wonder, though only fleetingly...if they think I am coming out of it okay.

"One of the 'little things,' and this is an understatement, that really almost irritates me, is the connection of a child and cancer being totally tragic to some people. You can tell in their tone. And for a quick (private) moment," Jayne says, *"I want to shriek: "She gave us life–kept us alive–kept us together gave each day some shape!' But instead I find myself looking probably pious or something and say, quietly, 'but Amy was a joy; she kept us going.'*

"[Still,] it is weird to hold all that joy and misery together in my mind," she says, speaking perhaps for both herself and her husband. *"Sometimes I think it wasn't so bad (Kenny is a stoic, completely non-hysterical and from a medical family, unlike mine) and then I almost want to trip myself up and stab out, 'It was just awful,' while I remember Amy blowing raspberries at us at three months. ... I also remember walking Amy around the old cemetery behind our house (it was near and I needed somewhere private to cry loudly–I couldn't do that at home and I couldn't go far because it still hurt to walk after Amy's birth–my pelvis was healing). I phoned a friend from work (of all people, and I called her before my parents and friends) and shrieked and cried from that cemetery.*

"I also remember leaving Kenny in the city hospital, which did do a fantastic job, after all...the night before his surgery. And [I remember] seeing him full of fear, and going back down and out to the tarmac where my friends were wheeling Amy up and down. Two of my oldest friends and Ken's mom. I couldn't hold his hand all day post–op either, as I had Amy to deal with.

"Now I feel old and worried. We are so financially strapped—we have not and probably never will recover from 18 months-to-two years of no income at all. And I wonder whether Kenny's cancer will recur. And as you know, every twinge is something coming back. But

on the other hand, which I always feel with this 'topic,' we are here, we are alive, Amy is a joy to us—true gorgeous joy and we're moving on. This year our garden might be good—so much died the summer Kenny was ill…and we've been busy since.

"Sometimes I think Kenny and I 'soldiered on' and pretended to each other, and kept the morale and chin up for so long that we became strangers to a degree, or were lacking some 'intimacy.' And even now—because we still cannot talk about cancer in the past tense—we are still in it and will be forever ensnared, I suppose. Even now we do not talk about those experiences that we had because our present and future is totally connected to all that."

This is what Jayne mostly said to me, shortly after I asked her to try and help me get a sense of how she and Kenny have put cancer "in its place." She didn't try to speak for him, in this instance. She was the spouse and caregiver (and new mom); not the patient. Turns out, though, that she didn't have to speak for him. Her words quite elegantly did the job for both. I'll not soon forget what she said about her family's bout with early, aggressive colon cancer. I'll not soon forget, either, the power of one comment she made to me: "This year our garden might be good."

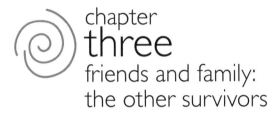

chapter
three
friends and family:
the other survivors

" " I t's not fair." Course it's not. Yet when I say I thought that
thought during the worst stages of my treatment, I wasn't
thinking only about sad-sack me. It was Paula I was thinking about,
who, yes, vowed to care for me "in sickness," but who, like me,
never thought the need would arise so soon. This was our sixth
year of marriage; not our 26th, nor 46th. Not fair.

For far too long Paula ran my life; she ran my bath. She ran my
treatment schedules; she cooked, blended, chopped, shopped and
looked for the light through all the dark. She took the tough phone
calls; she shuttled me to-and-fro the hospital wards and blood-draw
rooms that smelled, faintly, of disinfectant. Like a trainer guiding
a gimpy halfback to the sidelines, she'd sling her arm around me
when I was wobbly from fatigue, and lead me down the stairs
to the sunken radiation rooms. Other times at home, she played
bouncer—keeping a few energy-sapping souls from getting too-too
near to us, when it all seemed too exhausting. Post-op, sleeping
overnight in my room, she handled my urgent food-drink-bedpan
needs when the metal staples in my stomach were fresh—and when
a man in my condition needed the toughest advocate he could find.
When I got a little better, she was my lover again, though we were a
hundred times more careful than we'd ever been.

Through the worst of it, Paula won the big battles on my behalf, as my wife/partner/friend. And yet there was so little I could do, in that state, for her in return. I mouthed thank-yous; I told her that I loved her. Inside I vowed to try with everything I had to get stronger, to get better. For her and for me. Then, after a few hopeful scans and blood-test check-ups, once I started to believe I might actually be around a few years, I began to think about her circumstances: My wife deserved better. Still does. "It's not fair."

me, cancer, and geoff

One of the things I couldn't get from my wife, from Day One of diagnosis through Year Three follow-up, was black humor. Healing black humor. That was most often delivered by my best friend, for whom life wasn't fair either—ever since his mother died of cancer when he was 13. If Paula was my Rock, Geoff was my hard place.

Calling in from Chicago, while I'm still in shock-awe about a malignant tumor in my body, he says, "I got an idea. You can do a book; call it: *Me, Cancer, and Geoff.* Instead of a book about how you and your wife got through this together, it'll be a buddy book about how I helped you kick cancer. I'll be calling you every day; people aren't expecting that." Pause.

"You're sick," I say.

"I know," he says. "But I gotta ask you: Does this mean I'll have to do one of those Run-Walk things with you in five years?"

(Addendum: In fall, 2004, I invited Geoff, my friend for 33 years, to accompany me in the 5K, fund-raising "Snoopy Walks to End Colon Cancer," activists' event in Washington, D.C., in honor of "Peanuts" creator Charles M. Schulz, who died of colon cancer in 2000. Half expected Geoff to show up last-minute, clad in a zig-zag Charlie Brown sweater.)

go team [part I]

As anyone who's fought cancer knows, it's an understatement to say it helps to have help. Not just for physical demands, but for the longer-term, psychological ones as well. You're not alone in your hurt. We know that: Been there, felt that. We also think we know that because so much needs to be done, the sooner the patient can get back to "normal," the better.... But recovery isn't that simple. Especially when those closest to you have assumed multiple, integral roles in your daily life. At one point I remembered thinking, "How do I show I'm not so damn dependent?"

One of the first things I did, even before my surgery when I could neither handle stairs nor walk two blocks outside by myself, was push-ups. Not bolt-straight, military "Drop down and Gimme Fifty!" push-ups, but 10-to-20 pseudo-push-ups. "Girly" push-ups, Gov. Schwarzenegger might call 'em. I'd stand at the foot of the bed, or at the sturdy bathroom sink, take a step back, and do a dozen or more lean-to exercises, lowering, then slowly raising, my body from a measly, 60- or 75-degree angle back up to 90.

I wasn't going after biceps at this point: I was aiming for minimal maintenance of what muscle I had left. Also, I was trying to show my wife—my teammate—that each and every night, whether it actually helped or not, I would and could do something for myself.... Wanted her to see I had some strength left; wanted her to see I was determined to be more of a man again. I wanted her to know that she wasn't in this—no matter how she might have felt—alone.

Months later, when I was much, much stronger (but still wondering whether I was carrying half our marriage's "load"), I came across an apt passage from author Jeremy Geffen, M.D., an oncologist who wrote *The Journey Through Cancer*: "Remember that your spouse and family cannot meet all of your emotional needs. It is unfair and unwise to ask them to do so. You can help yourself, and them, by finding other places for support."

Note to self: Is now the time for me finally to knock on the door of the Colorado colon cancer support group's local chapter? Do they do push-ups in there?

do the math

Instead of doing push-ups, Shari Rogoff, 38, of Englewood, New Jersey, did the math. After caring for both her mother, who died of uterine cancer in 1999, and her father, who died of colon cancer in 2001at age 62, it came time for her to make a survivor's plan, rather early in life: "What's the best way for me to avoid getting cancer?" she asked. She admired greatly her dad's spirit and fight through then advanced stages of his disease; the fact that he'd even voted for taking powerful, radiation treatments near the end of his life. He did so, in hopes that "if I hang on, I might make it to the experimental trial of that ImClone." Genetically-speaking, she didn't much like the DNA she'd been dealt.

"I was told," she says, "not to worry about a colonoscopy till I was 49," she says. "That's 10 years down the road. It'd be the age at which my dad's cancer was diagnosed. But I told my doctor that's not good enough. Because if you do the math, and believe me, I did it, you'll figure that colon cancer cells can develop and hide in polyps for years before they're diagnosed. So I subtracted another 10 from my dad's age and made an appointment for a colonoscopy. I was 38. Sure enough, the doctor woke me from the twilight drugs and said, 'We found three polyps and took them out.' The next week, when the pathology report came back, my doctor called me and told me they were the kind that turn into cancer. I got lucky, and, literally, saved my ass.

"I was supposed to come back and get another colonoscopy in three years, but I wasn't satisfied with that. So the doctor recommended I come back for a repeat colonoscopy in two. I said, 'What would you do if I came back in one year for a follow-up?' He said,

'I'd give you a Valium and send you home.' But if I hadn't done the math," Rogoff says, "I would definitely have had colon cancer."

go team [part II]

At some of my worst times, physically, I was also blessed to have a seamless stream of close family members, flying to see me in San Francisco, all from Chicago. They came, one-at-a-time at pre-arranged times and weeks (to spread the total visit time) to help with my care; Mom, Dad, sister Beth (whose husband Howard initiated Sabbath prayers for me every Saturday, for months on the home-front). Out of my earshot they'd worked it all out with Paula: the details of who was coming when. I had no clue. But I knew I was never... alone. During these stretches I felt comforted, maybe a little wigged out, but as close to back-in-the-womb as a middle-aged, seriously diseased man could climb. With intimate, selfless support like this, I remember thinking, Could I actually consider myself "lucky?"

tag team

No way did Helen Lyman, at age 68, consider herself lucky during her colon cancer fight. For starters, she received a Stage 4 diagnosis; one that, at first, looked rather grim. "I had a lot of pain in the appendix; cancer was found; they took it out," she says, matter-of-factly. "I was fine. Then I [got] diverticulitis and was misdiagnosed: They gave me pain meds and I went on to China, where I was teaching for the State Department. The pain persisted, until they did a scope, and surgery and chemo...." Worse news followed, but she rebounded. "I'm not supposed to be around," she says, again matter-of-factly.

"Obviously, it's always a shock when you get the diagnosis," says her husband, Princeton Lyman, a State Department veteran and former U.S. ambassador to Nigeria and South Africa. "And

Helen's attitude was absolute determination to fight the disease. But you want to share that....

"Helen didn't want to be alone in the hospital," says Princeton, "because she was alone when she was told she had only a 15 percent chance of recovery. [What happened was] the oncologist had made his rounds late at night; and I was working and couldn't be there."

Adds the ambassador: "I don't listen to those statistics any longer—because that was devastating for us." The statistics said Helen should have died some years ago. These days, he says of his wife, "You don't tell someone how to feel. Helen got angry for a while, at the pain.... So sometimes I 'let her' feel discouraged. It's alright to let someone be a little angry."

a key de-stressor

Once the shock and anger fades, a patient's support team tends to get... analytical. Oftentimes the focus turns to: "Who is to blame for this disaster?" And, in many cases, rightly so. But over the long-term, over years of hoped-for survival, the patient and caregivers benefit more when they try to replace anger, negative energy or stress with more positive emotions. Admittedly, this is easier said, and written, than done. Especially with so many still-unknown links between the mind and body.

While stress is known to negatively affect our health in various ways, can it cause cancer? Can we blame it? "This is the era of stress causing everything in the world. It's very unfortunate," says Barrie Cassileth, Ph.D., director of Memorial Sloan-Kettering Cancer Center's integrative medicine unit in New York City and author of *Alternative Medicine Handbook: The Complete Reference Guide to Alternative and Complementary Therapies.* "There certainly is a mind-body link, but I don't think the mind causes cancer and I don't think the mind can cure it."

From this point on, if you believe Cassileth's take (and after interviewing her, I became a disciple) it becomes clear that stress-management—through music, DVDs, massage, tears or quiet talks—can be a worthy goal of patients, friends and family. Dealing with stress is no longer just a "to-do" to cross off one's list after yoga class. After all, as long as it's (undeniably) here, your goal and that of your caregiver(s) shifts a bit.

According to Cassileth, reactions to major health stresses tend to cause some fairly predictable, or automatic, behaviors.

Knowing now what to expect may help navigate them in the future:

◎ temporary denial

◎ connecting with loved ones

◎ imposing structure or order in a new setting or life phase

◎ connecting spiritually through prayer or meditation

◎ reaching out to others in need

feelings…

Sometimes it's just plain tough to reach out, on either side of the invisible wall that surrounds each newly diagnosed patient. That was how Judy Webster, then 56, of Omaha, Nebraska, felt (see pg. 63), when she literally tried to reach over to some folks she thought would understand her needs to reconnect, soon after her new diagnosis of colorectal cancer. "I didn't want to hurt my friends, who didn't know what to say…or how to act," Webster says.

"What I wanted to do was just go over there and hug my friend and hold her, and you couldn't do that either, because it makes people feel funny. So you have to be 'up'; you have to have hope and be strong for them. Because they don't want to see you weak. Just try to be strong for them, I guess." Which is one way to de-stress the circumstances, albeit not an easy way.

home alone

The patient from Wilmington, Sara-Jo Matthys, 46, didn't want me to take this the wrong way. During her first bout with breast cancer, in her early 40s, she was alone, but not totally alone. For we both knew, as cancer survivors who shared a mutual friend, that her marriage ended in divorce in the early 1990s, long before her diagnosis. "I got married way too young," she said. "I had just graduated college, at 22. He was an older guy, a photographer, and I got swept along."

By the time she was diagnosed and treated for breast cancer, however, she was 43 years old, and barely into a relationship. So when it came time to deal with the scare of her life, she had no husband or life partner to help her through the ordeal. "I did have a boyfriend at the time," she says. "He bailed out. He was there during the diagnosis, but left after a couple months. He told me 'I'm just really not a good caretaker.' So I guess he wasn't the man for me for whatever reason.

"Around that time, I remember thinking...'Am I gonna lose my breast? My hair? My boyfriend? Is he gonna care? Or be grossed out?' I became my sole support."

For most of her treatment, Sara-Jo was alone. She worked at her home-based consulting business; she often dragged herself to all manner of doctor and hospital appointments. Aging, infirm, parents, just one out-of-town sibling...two more reasons her friends were her last leg of support. (And her saving grace, she told me later.) But one weekend early in her treatment, a friend drove nine hours to spend two weeks with her and keep her company through a rough patch.

"I was crying for the entire weekend right after surgery," says Matthys. "I had problems with my [post-surgical] drains. My friend came to say things like: 'You're sooo negative. You've got to stop thinking about this stuff 24/7.'

"How could I not think that way? I realized then-and-there I didn't want to inflict this on someone else. If I wanted to cry myself to sleep, which I did a lot, then having someone sitting in the other room, freaking out, wasn't going to help me. There was nothing she could do for me. Unlike your family, I didn't feel I could be—or let her be—unconditional in our roles. I came to realize I didn't want to burden her. When it came time for me to get injections of Neupogen for 10 days straight, after treatment, I learned how to inject myself with a hypodermic syringe. And I know...it would have been different with a husband or boyfriend."

chemo by the bay

Thing about cancer is, nobody wants to be there: Not the patient; not his wife or family; not even his docs, sometimes, if we're all telling the truth here. And usually not his friends. They all have families and careers and wives or exes—and other friends, too. So it was surprising to me, amazing actually, when I realized maybe eight weeks into my ordeal, that a dozen, maybe even more, of my friends, were reaching out to me: physically, emotionally, prayerfully, financially, medically, even comically.

This was powerful stuff, to a midlife patient in crisis. Could relationships such as this, I wondered at times, actually help the chemo and radiation do its stuff? At one point I looked back and wrote:

"Easing into a leatherette La-Z-Boy in the UCSF infusion center, waiting for my blood work and for two friends to come by. (Farley's a San Fran local; Pete'll fly in from Denver for a few hours.) Suddenly I hear Paula say, 'Oh, my God, there's Brandy!'—meaning my grade-school friend who's joined by my high-school bud Jerry, which means we're having a surprise San Francisco-chemo-by-the-Bay party, only half of which I was expecting....

"Can't believe these guys pulled this one off—that with four wives and 13 kids among them, they were able to shuck their schedules, blow off clients, and see if they couldn't give me some old-style, are-we-ever-gonna-grow-up, ball-busting support. On a day I might not feel much like partying.

"For the occasion, Farley rents a 1450cc Harley (which Brandy falls off of while stopped at a stoplight); Pete raids the free (!) graham-crackers-and-apple-juice 'for patients only' pantry; and Jerry makes gross jokes about the rubber gloves he doesn't seem to want to take off.... I'm back in high school again, laughing my head off with old friends...till the drugs make me weak and the airport calls the boys home."

caregiver tips: what to say . . . and not to say

When you get news that cancer has hit someone close to home or work, here are some patient-tested guidelines to help keep the "care" in caregiver:

What to say:

- Useful information is welcome, but random stories of other cancer patients with sad—or happy—endings are not.
- Instead of: "Call me if there's anything I can do," let the patient know you'll be bringing something by. And when. For even the most widely used, genuine, offer has a glitch: A family in cancer crisis has no time to dole out chores. Get a solid idea for a good deed and simply do it.
- "I / we love you." (Can't hear that one enough.)
- "You don't need to call/write/e-mail back." Patients appreciate being let off the hook.
- "We've added you to our prayer circle." (Can't hear this one enough.)
- "I / we love you." (Told you we patients can't hear that one enough.)

What not to say:

- Before you ask a patient whether their type of cancer "runs in the family," you might first ask yourself: "I wonder how many times this question's been asked." Then consider: Even if it does run in the family, how exactly will this answer help the newly diagnosed patient feel or get better? (On the flip side, if there is no hereditary/genetic link, might this imply that the cancer patients did something to "cause" their cancer to develop?)
- If you say something from the *faux pas* file, apologize. But cancer patients get to say anything they want.
- Never tell a balding man who's losing his few survivors to chemo, "Well, there wasn't much there, anyway."
- "I know how you feel." You can't.

what to do . . . or not to do

What to do:

- You have a license to be angry. Feel free to use it...occasionally.
- Laughter is healing; silly joke gifts are not.
- Listen carefully; take notes for the patient and keep your comments simple. A gleam of acknowledgment goes a long way. A good go-to: "Just wanted to let you know that I'm thinking about you and praying for you."
- Acknowledge or grieve for what you've lost; give yourself/yourselves permission to forge ahead with new plans and dreams.
- Kiss a receptionist: Well, not literally. But when acting as advocate for a family member or friend, there's more to the role than coordinating docs, medicines, meals and insurance. That's why it pays, literally, to always ask—and jot down— the name(s) of those who help you along the way. The best receptionists and office-assistants can save a cancer patient time, money and discomfort. (They can also magically move your chart or results in front of a doctor's eyes much more quickly if they get to know you—and like you.) So spend the extra minute or two—no need to be cloying—each visit and try to wrangle the front-office worker onto your team.

What not to do:

- Don't give unsolicited self-help books, at first. The last thing a new cancer patient needs is to feel guilty about the stack of unread "How to Get Betters" beside the bed.
- Don't tell them how to feel. They may not want to play the 'glad' game, and instead might want to indulge in maudlin humor. It's their call.
- Don't be a drain. Keep those random horror stories, gloomy statistics, far, far away.
- Don't ignore your own needs. When was the you sense a shift from fatigue to despair or depression. last time you took a walk? Or spent quality time with...yourself? Don't feel guilty about caring for yourself as well as the patient.
- Don't be afraid to contact a support group or therapist if you sense a shift from fatigue to despair or depression.

caregiver solutions

Today, with about 12 million cancer survivors living in the U.S., the field of caregiving has moved beyond booming…to sprawling. Here are a few time-tested and respected places to find support for caregivers when you're feeling, at times, as if you've got nothing left to give:

- The National Coalition for Cancer Survivorship: the original grassroots advocacy and survival organization. **www.canceradvocacy.org 877-622-7937**

- National Family Caregivers Association **www.nfcacares.org 301-942-6430**

- Cancer Recovery Foundation of America: includes therapy-guided treatment sources and spiritual advice. **www.cancerrecovery.org 800-238-6479**

- *Today's Caregiver* magazine: **www.caregiver.com 800-829-2734**

chapter four
intimate matters: bedroom, bathroom, beyond

You hear a lot of medi-speak as a cancer patient. Too much, in fact. You forget a lot of it, too; your ears glaze over. Call it another coping mechanism. Yet there's one quote I haven't forgotten, nearly four years since a doctor spoke it. When I first heard those words, less than a month after diagnosis, I knew I had to write it down because it said something bizarre, and urgent, about the world I had unwillingly entered:

eight words you don't want to hear

"There I am, below ground, splayed out on a hard exam table in the UCSF radiation-therapy room, hospital-pajama bottoms pulled halfway down my crotch...when a senior member of the radiation/oncology team addresses a younger doctor after viewing my simulation—the precise position I will be in when radiation beams will enter my body. He uses eight words: 'The penis is going to have a reaction.' In other words, the penis (which would be mine) will very likely develop a severe sunburn of sorts, over six weeks of absorbing adjacent, anti-cancer radiation waves. Note to self: 'Prepare.'"

the power of touch

What I didn't want, despite all the kind offers sent my way, was anybody to touch me after my surgery; after being prepped, poked, anal-probed, radiated, carved, rerouted, stapled together, benumbed, and finally, wheelchair-discharged. What I didn't want was anybody to touch me...including, at times, my wife. Not a healthful situation, it would seem, after all she had done for me over six, seven, nine months' time.

Point is, I remember thinking this at first while Paula was having a "housecall" massage, soon after her scoliosis-addled back reared up and brought her down. I wasn't envious of the soothing, oil-infused, tender care she was receiving in the room next door. Nor was I jealous that the massage therapist was a guy. (Alright, maybe a touch jealous of that.) I simply knew I'd rather be all by my lonesome, near-wretching with chemo-nausea...staring at a tepid bowl of macaroni and cheddar while watching ESPN baseball...than having some soft-talking masseuse pressing in on my body with his scrubbed-pink, über-trained fingertips and thumbs...digging all in and his palms providing punctuation. Me? I was just fine 15 feet from him—feeling post-traumatic-heck-with-em. I was living largely horizontal, in a state 40 pounds lighter than when I started this treatment gig. Point is, as the able-bodied fans stood up and took a seventh-inning stretch on TV, I improvised and rolled over onto my side. And wondered whether I was building a shell of sorts around me.

the power of gynecological touch

In spring, 2001, William Fuller, M.D., then-chairman of Obstetrics and Gynecology at Health One's Presbyterian-St. Luke's Hospital in Denver, who's delivered more than 5,000 babies in over 20 years of practice, pulls me aside and tells me that, because of the stories I've written about my cancer and my misdiagnosis, he is changing

the power of tumescence

When you're fighting for your life, it's not surprising to find the importance of orgasm isn't, well, as important as it was before. That's not to say sex isn't important; it's more a sad fact of survivor reality.

In my case, after hearing from three different doctors that I may lose some or all of my "powers of erection" after tricky colorectal surgery that would take place in part near my prostate gland, I remember feeling, with my wife at my side, both embarrassed and resigned: "Okay...then..., maybe it's Viagra for life." With an emphasis on "for life."

It's a deal I was prepared to make, to exit my surgery cancer-free. (It's also not as if I had a bushel of options.) In order to excise a large, Stage III tumor embedded in and around the rectum, the surgeons at University of California-San Francisco's Moffitt Hospital were going to have to be both aggressive and unusually sensitive— sensitive, that is, to all sorts of nerves bundled near my prostate and perineum (beneath the sub-dermal section from scrotum to anus) that have lots to do with how erections form...and perform. (For women, Ob-Gyns have informed me, orgasmic waves happen here....)

Looking back, I'd never call myself "lucky" after what I'd faced at a relatively young age—43—and after enduring a missed diagnosis or three. But I consider myself extremely fortunate in one regard: Thanks to the profuse skill (plus experimental, nerve-tracking, nerve-sparing technique) of surgeons Welton and Carroll, I can forthrightly report that at 46, I've yet to require the "oomph" services of such esteemed pharmaceuticals as Levitra, Viagra or Cialis. The docs got my cancer out, and in expertly doing so saved my innate powers of...tumescence.

how he practices medicine. He will now add digital (rectal) exams to the standard workup in his patients' checkups if they are over age 40 or at risk for colorectal cancer. For many women, these digital exams had been optional—they simply weren't thought of as automatic Ob-Gyn terrain. This means, in part, the publicity of my case will help, if not immediately save lives, then at least improve the future sex lives of an untold number of Dr. Fuller's patients—and those of their partners.

am i normal, yet?

When is sex not quite sex? One answer, according to Terry Real, a marital and family therapist in Cambridge, Massachusetts, and author of *The New Rules of Marriage,* is: when people are feeling undue pressures about major life events. These pressures, which arise during financial upheavals and recovery from such major illnesses as heart attack and cancer, can lead to unexpected and uncomfortable moments in bed. Even between eager, compatible sex partners.

"His nerves may cause him to seek sex when all he really wants is reassurance or some support from his partner," Real explained to me. "It's just that he might find it easier to reach out for that support under the covers late at night rather than in the kitchen, face-to-face…. He may want to talk, but what he knows to do is grab her in bed."

---

sex and my cancer (part I)

Early on in my treatment, I had a mini-confessional:

"Haven't yet poked around the standard patient Websites about sex and colon cancer…," I reported. "Here's what I know so far: In one month of being a colon-cancer patient, I've had sex twice; once what I would term successfully. The other time, well, that's what I know about sex and my cancer."

"Grab" instead of talk? Guilty as charged. This was, at times, undeniably true in my case, and, I'm guessing, in countless others'. We may not often say it, but I will here: As mind/body-damaged survivors, we may want so badly to prove we're back to "normal," that we can hardly help using sex as a crutch. Makes it difficult, then, for maybe the first six months to a year post-op, to consider sex a playful event. Which is not to say we shouldn't have it. Or enjoy it. Real and his therapist colleagues aren't preaching that: They are looking instead to lead us to acknowledging weighty feelings of inadequacy and (possibly misplaced) fears of mortality. Then, it's hoped, we can finally relax into sex once again.

sexological, oncological gynecology

Back before cancer put a crimp in my sex life, I discovered one "hot" new way to have better sex: What happened was, *Glamour* magazine hired me to write an article about new "lust lotions" women were trying out (under doctor supervision), to see if Viagra-type drugs, or creams, might work for them. Nice work.

The theory was similar to how men's erection drugs work, except that the lotions would be applied by hand, not popped in pill form.

---

sex and my cancer (part II)

Less than two months after diagnosis you could say I was tired; you could also say I was fried:

"Wondering, in bed, how long it will take for the barbecued, irradiated skin on my package to return to normal color and texture…. Finding that having an erection and doing something pleasurable with it hurts in such odd, frightening ways in the first weeks after radiation treatment…that it makes you think twice about having an erection and doing something pleasurable with it."

The goal: to boost blood flow to the vagina and clitoris in order to increase female sexual arousal or orgasms. One company, Vivus, even received a patent for such a specific, hormone-based cream. In researching these drugs, I learned a key lesson in female anatomy: the clitoris, like the penis, is much larger than it may at first appear. In fact the primary female sex organ contains countless bundles of nerves, arteries, veins and capillaries—a whole network of potential for pleasure. These nerves and vessels run beneath the clitoral (or erectile) shaft and spread both inward, toward the rectum, and outward, toward the thighs. Instead of a mere "pea-shaped organ," then, the clitoris can be described (depending upon the gynecologist doing the describing) as a longer, stronger, "inverted Y-shaped organ," in which the tongs of the "Y," or the pea-pods if you will, reach into the groin, well beyond the vagina.

The reason I'm recalling all this now is because I received a recent e-mail from a fellow-colon cancer survivor who happened to be female. And whose surgery happened to have some unfortunate Ob-Gyn complications:

"I'm trying to be active," Laurie B. said. "I can't do walking very well, as the radiation gave me second- and third-degree burns. I have had to accept a new normal.... And because of my treatments, as soon as I put food in my mouth I have to find the bathroom....

"That's just part of it," she added. "But I've been lucky. I had a three-year colonoscopy last week; it was clean, NED [no evidence of disease]. But life changes and there I am, four days later [with], orangutan bottom. When I walk too far, it goes to bleeding.

"The radiation took away all the soft tissue," Laurie explained, comparing her rectal cancer treatment to mine. [Except that her surgical side effects seemed to affect some spinal nerves as well; and are more feminine.] "I have to be dilated, because the rectum-to-sphincter [tissue] tries to shrink. It's like sitting on an open sore. I was also damaged vaginally: The gynecologist has to

sex and my cancer (part III)

So there I am, a few weeks after surgery—more than three, but who's counting?—I'm fooling around in bed with Paula, and it feels like high school fooling-around-in-bed….Because, honestly, I don't know what will happen...on my side of the bed...if we keep this up. Fact is...plumbing's been shut off for a while. Lotsa hands, more than usual, it seems. And I'm not thinking about baseball or the Queen Mother. I'm thinking, for a few seconds at least, about the doctor who warned me that I might be Viagra-dependent...for a while. For a long while.

Maybe for decades...but...not...now...."First time since surgery," I'm thinking, feeling a lot like in high school right now, with lotsa hands... and an odd, resurgent, genital-tickle-toward-inevitability...and a rhythmic pumping in the erection that almost wasn't...hold on...on the verge...of bringing unfamiliar groans of pleasure.

Feels so good I feel like shouting but I don't. Instead I'll just write about it, quietly, in the pages of a nationally published book. And maybe take a nap.

use a pediatric instrument to examine me. I had a reversal (of a stoma) on September 10, 2001; now they want to put the colostomy back on."

And I was worried, not too long ago, about a possible future need to simply swallow some Cialis for better sex.

trick faq?

A story in *GQ* magazine—arguably the modern metrosexual man's embodiment of fashion and style in print—once asked a simple question: "What is a man's most powerful sex organ? The answer is the brain."

It went on: "What, then, is a man's second most powerful sex organ? The answer is the skin."

Point is, skipping the technicalities: No matter what happens, temporarily or more permanently, to a cancer patient's crotch—as a result of chemotherapy, radiation or surgery—there's a lot left to play with; a lot left to enjoy.

a friend wants to know...

"Do you think about cancer every day?" a friend writes, a friend who doesn't really know my whole story, but who wants to know more.

"Yes," I answer, "in part because they took out my colon during surgery...." (Hope I didn't sound angry when answering him, 'cause it's been five or six months since the operation.) "Yes," in other words, because I now have a handicap. "Yes," because I'm now what the gastro-cancer health professionals call, an "ostomate." There's colostomy, where the colon gets rerouted through the torso; and ileostomy, where the small intestine is what's left. That's me. Not a major handicap, some would say—compared with the likes of Stephen Hawking or what Christopher Reeve endured. But as one of the vast minority (approximately 15 percent) of colorectal cancer patients who sacrificed a bowel or rectum in order to become cancer-free, I can't help but think about cancer two, three, maybe four brief times a day—when I have to use the bathroom in an unconventional way; when I empty the contents of my polyethylene pouch into the toilet, before flushing, before washing my hands (like everybody else), and before going back on the other side of the bathroom door...into the world where I won't think about cancer, least for a while.

can abs be too strong?

They didn't warn my cancer-stricken pal beforehand. Maybe because they didn't know. When young Martin (not his real name), all of 35, found out he was slated to have a temporary ileostomy diverted through his lower torso during rectal cancer surgery, he did a smart thing. He took some time and tried to get into shape for the operation. Rowing machine, swimming, ab work: the guy did his homework.

Problem was, after the surgery (successful!) to remove his cancer, his stoma didn't function properly. In fact it hardly functioned at all. No light through the end of the tunnel. Which caused him extreme, lose-major-sleep pain and misery, as all sorts of undue pressure was being exerted on a section of small intestine that was not working. For unknown reasons (including possible surgical error), it was not allowing food to pass out of the body, through the temporary and new-fashioned anus, while the rest of his digestive tract healed. They said it might take six-to-eight weeks. Trouble was, Martin had abs. Honest-to-goodness abs, bordering on six-pack; earned from years of sustained, teeth-clenching ab exercises. And yet, unfortunately for him, the muscularity of the six-pack seemingly bunched up around the detoured small intestine and apparently pinched it shut, like a crimp in a garden hose you left out all winter. (His ileostomy, like most, was threaded through the ab muscles and out the lower torso.) Next time, he and his family vowed—though they hope to heavens they'll never see a next time—he'll let himself get a bit more squidgy in and around the middle. For "health" reasons; just to be safe.

the resection: the healing colon

Most people who have colon cancer, it bears repeating, don't end up with a permanent colostomy. In truth, fewer than 20 percent face this type of digestive-disease-related disfigurement. In the hospital there's a cutting out of diseased colon, maybe 6 inches, maybe a foot and a half (of the total five to six feet) or more (in my case the whole organ). Then comes "resection," which means stitching together of the two remaining sections that have been rendered "open" during the surgery. In general, in approximately 20 percent of colon cancer surgeries, the patient's bowel habits are noticeably and at times frustratingly affected.

In the best case scenario...resection that is done during first surgery...all intestines wake up and start working within 24-to-48 hours. A clean resection. But with cancer, as we've seen, things don't always go cleanly. Depending upon which portion(s) of the colon were removed, patients often have to adjust to a new schedule of bowel movements, replete with new habits.

Sometimes survivors will heal on schedule, yet never feel as if their bowels are quite emptied. Other times frequency (three times a day instead of one) or consistency of stools change markedly. (With less colon in place, there's less organ tissue with which to remove water from your waste.) There's no doubt a nurse will review all this with you—if she or he hasn't already—before your discharge from the hospital. You may even be warned that you'll need to "retrain yourself" a bit on going to the toilet. But it's a tough thing to talk about—taking a dump, anew. It's a tough thing to even want to talk about.

the symptoms, second time around

Most of us know the Big Five, the warning signs of colorectal cancer: 1] abdominal cramping; 2] blood in the stool or toilet; 3] rectal bleeding; 4] thinning stools; and 5] "false" urges to have a bowel movement. But we also know early stage colon cancer may be masked by other conditions (constipation, inflammatory bowel disease). So, besides tracking your CEA (carcinoembryonic antigen) test two or three times per year, anyone especially concerned about recurrence may want to talk with their oncologist about using at-home stool or fecal-occult blood tests.

the endorsement: the bag

It is not exactly pretty; it is something I am not exactly proud of. The bag I now wear, along with thousands of other colorectal-cancer survivors, is a flesh-colored, polyethylene utensil not that different in shape or appearance from a flattened, up side-down, old-fashioned milk bottle, the kind you see at carnivals and county fairs—"Three throws for a dollar...knock 'em off the table!"

The bag is two fists tall or thereabouts, reaching, as I stand, from next to my navel to the glans of my (nonerect) penis. The bag, also called "the pouch" by ostomy experts, is emptied three times a day and at bedtime and changed every three days or so. Featuring two openings—one that attaches to my lower torso with skin-friendly adhesives, the other that empties into the toilet and clips shut—the bag is a lot better alternative than an adult diaper, I'd say; others might say, cynically, "That Depends." I would not however say that. For the bag is hidden under boxers and is airtight-water-tight-hygienic. Even as it is not exactly attractive.

The tests are portable, private, and now over-the-counter. They also inadvertently turn your toilet into a forensic device, as you hunt "invisible" intestinal blood in the privacy of your bathroom. By simply taking a smear of stool from tissue (using a gloved hand if you prefer) and sending the wrapped plastic swab-utensils to the lab, survivors can rather easily add an extra layer of prevention and assurance to their year-round, anti-cancer efforts. There are even newer, more high-tech tests, such as those made by the Exact Sciences Corporation, which use genetic markers to screen bowel movements for early signs of colorectal cancer. Big plus: the specimen "collections" are made in the privacy of your own home. (for more information, check: Exactsciences.com)

the non-endorsement: the bag

Accidents will happen. In the notable, 1997 nonfiction book *Man-to-Man*, author and publishing exec Michael Korda talks about how, leading up to his diagnosis of prostate cancer, he dealt with the fact that his urogenital works—bladder/prostate/penis—were in trouble. He knew this in part because he had started charting particular pedestrian pathways—en route to his office everyday—through and around parking lots in Midtown Manhattan, so he could easily reach the rare, open-to-public bathrooms, before his bladder gave out from urgency and inflammation. He was a 60-year-old man who felt older.

In my case, my ostomy bags have leaked five or six times over nearly four years. Twice, minor leaks followed extended airplane trips, coincidentally or not (maybe the cabin pressure?). Two more times bags have pulled partly away following unexpected athletic-type moves (not on playing fields or golf courses, but in an office and outside next to a parking lot). They've more admirably survived ski mountain falls, swimming pools, hot tubs (though not recommended for long stretches of time), twice-weekly mountain bike rides, a 10-K road race at altitude, and an untold number of a two-year-old's climbing-on-Daddy maneuvers. Sure, stuff happens. But there's usually an early warning, a tension signal-on-skin that signals the wearer to head to the john for repairs. And it doesn't happen nearly as frequently as I, or my fellow "ostomates," would have thought (www.ostomy.org).

wise words: valuable lessons from the surgical ward front lines

After 20 years of caring for colorectal cancer patients, most of whom have had major surgery, Susan Barbour, R.N., of the University of California-San Francisco, is a human Website/encyclopedia of sorts when it comes to a survivor's most personal feelings. She counseled me before and after my surgery, taught me how to live with an ileostomy; and somehow I felt we would always share a strong, if odd, connection. Sure enough, when I contacted her to help with this chapter, it felt as if we'd only been "apart" for a few months. Life-saving surgery does have a way of bringing people...closer.

"Ostomy issues are so loaded in our society," she says. "If the child, spouse or friend of a patient has issues with it, those issues come through to the patient. If you're uncomfortable with it, it comes through. I'll often ask the spouse direct questions if I have a feeling [there's discomfort there]. We go talk in the hallway; I try to normalize it."

Regarding the bathroom inevitables, Barbour says, "Gloves— people ask if they should wear gloves to change the bag. I say, 'Do you wear gloves when you go? When you change a baby's diaper?' It's kind of the same thing. That's something everybody asks, gloves. I downplay that. I'm a minimalist. Some nurses come in with a suitcase full of supplies, gizmos.

"Sometimes family members want to do a lot, to help, change it. I say, okay, but I find out what the patient wants. I force the issue—I make sure the partner sees it in the hospital, in a supportive environment. I'll show the stoma to them. One woman thought her stoma was temporary, so she put off intimacy with her husband—she didn't want him to see it. It turned out, after a year and a half, to be a permanent stoma. They had no sex for a year and a half. Another couple, I had a lesbian couple, they were in their 60s: The patient was concerned with the stoma; that her partner wouldn't like her as much. I tell them the patient needs to believe the partner when they say, 'I love you and don't care.' I'd say 90 percent (of partners) don't care.... But some people get compulsive with it."

In rapid-fire succession, nurse Barbour shared a handful of other insights, providing answers to colorectal questions I didn't know I had: "Some of the right things to say, to patients after surgery are: 'How are you doing? You look terrific.' When it comes to farts [in which gas from the small intestine rushes into the bag, briefly, instead of out of the usual orifice], I tell patients/partners to acknowledge them. Humor helps make light. 'Your stoma's talking to me....' It's worse to ignore them.

"As for intimacy, the partner often feels like they will hurt them. It's up to me to let them know they won't. Some people are terrified of hurting the patient, from just hugging, or anything physical. I had this [one] couple, in which stomach stroking was part of their routine. It was integrated into their foreplay. The partner was asking what to do? I said, 'Move along; you have the whole other side.'

"I might push people sometimes to get together, to talk and learn about the stoma [stuff]. Some people think it's temporary, but you never know when it's over. You don't want to let a piece of intestine on the outside get between them."

personal questions—and answers

Of all that's wrong with the Internet, one of the things that's right about it is how quickly it can offer—and deliver—answers to some of the most personal questions a person might have. Including questions of medically-affected sex, reproduction, elimination (as in the other kind of toiletry) and communication (as in therapy, psycho- or marital). Here are four top-notch places to turn when you don't quite have the right person available, right there next to you, to answer a few, or more, questions of urgency. Rest assured: These folks have Heard it All Before.

1. American Association for Marital and Family Therapy (AAMFT), Alexandria, VA 703-838-9808
In 20-plus years of practicing medical journalism, I've attended dozens if not hundreds of seminars, conferences and press conferences at which doctors or other health professionals have gathered to find or pitch solutions to our mind/body ills. I've also found, over the years, that the AAMFT annual meetings offer incredibly sound, practical, helpful advice to patients, clients, and couples in need of short- or long-term therapy (even when they aren't aware they need therapy). Though the annual meetings aren't open to the public, the AAMFT Website is. It can help match therapists and clients nationwide, in a snap. **www.AAMFT.org**

2. National Coalition for Cancer Survivorship (NCCS), Silver Spring, MD 877-622-7937 (toll-free) www.canceradvocacy.org
After the surgery, after the treatment, after all the hands-on help, here's a safe, scientifically sound place to go to connect with those interested in guiding you through the next phase of healing. Particularly helpful when you're more alone than you're used to being (and when your caregiver, perhaps, needs a little time off).

3. United Ostomy Association (UOA), Irvine, CA 800-826-0826 www.ostomy.org
The group, with its invaluable chat-lines, comprising specialized nurses, doctors, therapists and online patient advocates, tells it absolutely Like It Is. A major source of stress-relief to those who are dealing with colostomy, ileostomy or urostomy (urological stomas) issues for the first, or follow-up, times.

4. Intimate Partners by Maggie Scarf (Ballantine Books, 1988)
No Website needed, no doctors, no nurses, no cancer focus. Merely the best book I've ever read about getting closer to someone you love. It also offers staggeringly clear reasons why it is so difficult for husband and wife, boyfriend-girlfriend, or partner and partner, to connect at the highest, most significant, levels. It's got sex, psychology, infidelity, plus case studies. Bonus: Written by a writer, not a psychotherapist. **www.randomhouse.com or online booksellers such as bn.com.**

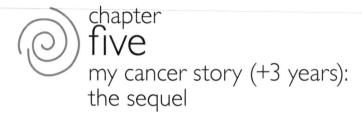

chapter five
my cancer story (+3 years): the sequel

re-intro, re-entry

Two years since diagnosis, and I am cancer-free. Don't call myself a survivor...yet; feels too early. Don't call myself a "warrior," either. That's for the charity-fund appeal and pink-ribbon ad-campaign writers. But I've taken nine months of treatment ("We're gonna pound you," my radiation doc said); recovered from life-saving surgery with most of my body intact ("Don't stop cutting till you see the table," my colorectal surgeon said [in jest]); adopted a child; and I have started hugging my family and friends a bit harder.

Call me middle-aged guy in remission—make that recovery—because the way I see it, remission only means temporary absence of disease. Call me healthy but wary. Been bouncing back and forth from the U.S. to London, where [my wife] Paula is once again working as associate producer on the *Harry Potter* films. Been writing again, even some new kinds of stuff for a documentary I'm trying to get made. Been getting used to getting cancer behind me, even if it'll always seem ahead of me. Also been getting used to being a new dad, to giving all sorts of care at all hours to Baby Josh, kind of like Paula did for me. Still don't feel, though, that beating advanced colon cancer has made me "a better man." Even if I am, I've noticed, more apt to sign off letters, cards, and notes with "love."

pulp friction

...Whirrrr-chop-chop-vrruuuuuuuhhhh!!! Got a juicer the other week, a bona fide institutional kind that weighs a ton, cost nearly $300, and grinds the goodness out of pretty much anything that grows on trees or out of the ground. *Vruhhhh-chop.* There's no scientific proof of freshly extracted juice adding 6.2 years to my life or anything; just advice from a good friend from Tulsa and a reasoned attempt to keep things that shouldn't be growing inside me from growing inside me.

race for my cure

SCENE: EXTERIOR: Glinting, early-a.m., late-spring sun, Boulder, Colorado. Heli-cam ESTABLISHING SHOT, rolls east over the Foothills of the Rockies, panning over thousands of Lycra-clad runners (and walkers) and civilian-dressed road race officials milling about, near the intersection of 30th Street and Iris Ave., near the STARTING LINE of the 26th Annual Bolder Boulder 10K race…. Police barricades and scores of port-a-potties are lined up all along the staging areas leading to the pushoff point. PUSH shot of runner awkwardly trying to pin race number on to T-shirt with safety pins….

EXTERIOR: CLOSE-UP ON AUTHOR, ME, 46-year-old colon cancer survivor, clad in bicycle shorts, T-shirt, sunglasses, new New Balance 860 running shoes… walking alone, slowly, toward start, one of 44,000 people who would enter the race this day. Tightening the Velcro straps on my warning/orange mesh jersey/vest—the one I'm wearing not for colon cancer aware-ness, but so my wife might find me during the run amid tens of thousands of non-survivors….

CUT TO: Rows of nervous runners moving slowly toward the starting line, like slaughterhouse cattle, only better dressed, and with lots less fat on their bones….

CLOSE-UP: *MACRO on my right leg, and my right hand, grabbing the instep and top of my right foot. Bending back the foot—and knee— in a faux stretch that I'm doing mostly because everyone else is doing it. I'm a part-time runner, not a stud. I'm stretching to pass the time till the starter's gun goes off, not really to prevent the pain and fatigue I'll soon feel.*

Wondering, now, with fewer than five minutes till my "wave" starts the race, whether I've trained long-and-hard enough for a 6.2-mile run... at altitude. Knowing that I've spent six weeks or so training; but that I also don't expect to set any speed records this morning. My main goal: to finish. My second goal: to finish in less than an hour. (I'd clocked the race at 53 minutes back in 1999, pre-diagnosis.) Gun goes off. We start....

Lagging in the first mile, it seems, because I keep looking for the first water or Gatorade station stop.... Thirsty already; heavy legged. Gaining ground and speed in mile 3; especially after seeing Paula and Joshua, waiting patiently—and waving wildly—from in back of the Moe's Bagels shop, not 35 yards away.... I have my own cheeering section, I'm thinking, which translates to a short boost of energy to crest the hill on 13th Street....

Heading out of mile 5 and toward the home stretch on Folsom (toward the University of Colorado Buffaloes football stadium), and cursing the last hill that tries to Slow Us Down... realizing that I'm going to finish the race. Without stopping. Not a marathon, but enough. Six point two miles...in 63 minutes. Not learning until a few weeks later that my place in said race was 17, 601 out of 44,000 or so who entered. So I didn't finish a sub-60 10-K, but I did run a "huge" race, in the top half of the field...in a time that was only 8 minutes slower than Frank Shorter, former Olympic marathon gold medalist. So what if he's in his 50s now? So what if he's a bit injured? I was still close to him (sort of). And maybe it doesn't much matter about the time. I trained, and finished, and learned. This ain't no Olympic trial. This is a colorectal cancer patient's attempt to take back his life, in one small way, three years after surgery. To blend in, literally, with the masses. And to run like I meant it, if only for today; if only for a short while....

SYNOPSIS: Training for a 10-K—running 8-10 miles a week, helps take one's mind off of "being a cancer patient." In my case, I became a runner again, if only for 63 minutes. In my case, the run helped me turn a corner on the disease aftermath, to help place it, frame it, more personally in my past. I could be, for an hour again, "one" with the masses, the (seemingly) healthy masses.

---

cheeseburger in paradise

"You ever get ticked at me that you ate healthy all those years, and I didn't..." asks Geoff on a rare day of candor-studded best-friend banter, "and you got cancer?" Truth is, I don't get ticked at Geoff for that; I actually worry about his health. And he is allowed to say stuff like this, we agree, because his mom died of cancer when he was 13 (and his dad, of diabetes complications, three years later). Have another bacon-cheese, Pal-o-mine.

---

celebrity and my cancer

Walking down skinny England's Lane, six weeks post-treatment, passing by a suitably Brit street sign: DEAD SLOW PLEASE—CHILDREN. Eyeing a guy wearing, of all things on a warm day, a red beret. Thinking I wouldn't bug the guy in New York or L. A., but this is London for chrissakes, and he isn't exactly blending in. I introduce myself to Tim Burton, without going googly or mentioning *Beetlejuice*, and end up inviting him to the premiere of *Harry Potter*. Then

I speed-dial Paula to warn her what I've done without checking with any Warner Bros. honchos.

"You've lost your filter," she says. Meaning I'll say pretty much anything I want these days, to pretty much anybody. Even to a guy who had the gall to remake *Planet of the Apes* with Marky Frickin' Mark.

"he's livin'"

[Excerpt from Paula's journal]

Back in England, I find I'm living with a forty-four-year-old teenager. Curt won't be where he doesn't want to be; or with whom he doesn't want to be with. He's spontaneous and seizing the moment, not wasting time with small talk, pretending he's interested. He went to a play on a whim on Friday...*Rent* (again)...with some college kids he didn't know who had an extra cheap ticket to spare. He ran into them in Leicester Square. I tell him I was worried. Couldn't reach him for hours. "I'm livin'!" he said, and thank God he is.

---

words you don't want to hear

"...She will be cremated today after the medical specialists learn what they can to assist other warriors against cancer."—E-mail from a friend, about another friend, on a day I wasn't planning to think about my cancer. Much.

words you want to hear

"I recently read your articles this spring and was compelled to write to you to express how I was moved by your story and your writing. I will keep you in my prayers. If there is anything I can provide from my meager life in the Midwest, please don't hesitate to contact me. Very Truly Yours, Chris Jensen" Didn't contact him; he provided it anyway.

somebody else's trouble

Every other Thursday, when I read the BBC.co.uk series by science writer Ivan Noble, about the malignant "tumour" that's found a home in his skull, I...read...every...word...incredibly...slowly. More slowly, perhaps, than anything I've ever read on my crappy Apple laptop. As if by doing so, I'm showing this guy in his mid-thirties—newly married with a baby daughter for God's sake—some extra respect. Or by my doing so maybe his "fast-growing" tumor will somehow grow more slowly. Because, as he says, he doesn't expect it to go away anytime soon. Not to compare, but I heard the word "curable" from at least one doctor during my diagnosis.

Noble heard no such thing from his esteemed neurosurgeon. "There are no good brain tumours to have, [the neurosurgeon] said, but if there were, mine would not be one of them." [postscript: Noble died in early 2005.]

new lang syne

12/27/02
TO: Chris and Monica
FROM: curtpmail@aol.com

dear monica and chris,

i went skating the other day, skated on the same rink i skated on two years ago this week, when i found out i had cancer....

i went skating the other day, skated with the same friend i skated with two years ago in boulder, the one i didn't have the strength to tell that awful day i just found out i had colon cancer....

i went skating the other day; did laps around the rink one way, then the other, while watching a mom with her 2-year-old and his double runners—double runners that didn't seem to be working very well.

i went skating the other day, as a new dad with clean CT scans....

i went skating the other day, thinking about Joshua joining me next year on that rink in Colorado; thinking about Paula who will be there worrying if he's going too fast around the corners, and I'll be thinking, "all's pretty much right with the world," thanks to good doctors, truly great friends like you, and some powerful, prayerful, medicine.

i went skating the other day, and this time the Christmas tunes didn't sound tinny, false, taped: this time they echoed off the ice and into my ears, into my heart.

now, everybody off the damn ice, so they can scrape it...clean it...and let everybody start over...doncha' know?

happy new year, guys, to you and your amazing family,

love, curt

---

three times a year

[Excerpt from Paula's journal]

I'm in a lot better place now, I guess because it's January. Next scans aren't till the end of April. That's because Dr. [Allen] Cohn says, "every three to four months (for the first two years after surgery, then every six)." And Curt's figured out, if we stretch it out till four, that's one less per year, plus less radiation.

I find myself now living my life with this benchmark. So far relieved, and filled with joy, but as the weeks pass, feeling the dread that so slowly creeps up on me, as the next trip home gets closer. When we sit in the oncologist's office, trying to anticipate and read into his every expression...hearts-are-racing...then learning he hasn't read them yet; will be right back....Trying to hear the pace of his footsteps as he returns to see if they will give me any insight as to the news about to be delivered. Do we get to continue our lives as they are—so full of love and joy, and our new baby, Joshua...or do we put on our gear again and go into the fire and fight for life?

as a jaybird

One thing I've noticed: Ever since cancer, ever since surgery, ever since I've owned a post-op stoma protruding ever so slightly from my torso, I don't flit about the house so often as I used to, naked.

my adoption story

You don't enter the world of adoption lightly. But in the summer of '96, after Paula almost died following an ectopic pregnancy that exploded, sort of, into her uterine insides, where some nasty arteries reside and where she internally bled quarts of blood for way too long before they figured out why her blood pressure had dropped to "0" ...we thought of it.

No, you don't enter the world of adoption lightly, so we have been in it heavily now, for two years running. And we have a son who wasn't born when I had my Big Run with colorectal cancer, and what am I going to tell him about it, not yet sure. Yet when he sees me in the shower wearing a Band Aid-colored bag on my lower torso, he's gonna ask eventually, so I will tell him what makes sense, what is true, along with the fact that were it not for my cancer, or Paula's ectopic, we may not have found Joshua Daniel, ever.

false alarm?

Waking on a cold morning, early winter, with a twinge astride my right testicle that ranges from groin to lower torso...uh-oh. Feels a little like a groin pull, but higher, and connected to the dull, lingering pains I feel in my lower abdomen when I do push-ups or other ab work (not that I do a lot of "ab work"). Surgery scar tissue, maybe, or worse? Make a note to ask about this pain at the next CT-scan checkup in two months.

the fire this time

"You smell something burning?" Paula says [July '02]. "You see the fire out there?" Hard to believe, hard to miss, but after three years of trying to get pregnant, and two years of trying to adopt, we finally bring our seven-month-old baby home from his poverty-ravaged Guatemala...and the neighborhood's nearly on fire.

Fewer than five hours after landing, on Josh's first night in the U.S., without warning, a Colorado wildfire erupts and crawls down the nearby foothills toward Wonderland Lake—and our backyard. "Unfrickin' believable," I'm thinking from the upstairs back bedroom window, "it's not burning itself out..." Instead, it's looking like molten lava moving over drought-starved grasses. Phone rings, we pick up. Friends up the road, forced out of their home. They're on the way over. Paula's in bed with Joshua, trying to let him sleep....

Phone rings again later; I pick up. "You are being advised to evacuate...." recorded message from the sheriff's office drones. It's 2:00 am. and we're haphazardly packing photos and bags furiously...aided by Nancy, Cory, Amelia, and Aidan and their Lab/ Rhodesian Ridgeback puppy that doesn't have a clue. No time to ponder the tragicomic timing—"Do we take the [big] wedding photo or the album??"—as the next chapter of our storybook life unfolds. We stay put. I stay up until 4:30 a.m. Next day we learn 400 acres got torched; nobody got killed; our property got a free pass....Welcome home, Son.

sex and my cancer

Viagra this, Viagra that. Didn't think, when I was fighting cancer so fiercely, that it would have made a huge deal if I had come out of surgery okay but learned I'd be Viagra-dependent for life. I was flat-out wrong (and glad I had crack surgeons). Spontaneous sex is thrilling, more so when you realize you nearly lost the chance to have it. Even so, to come clean, I don't have it nearly as often as I used to: The twice-a-week standard I've seen quoted so often hasn't applied to me or my partner, if she doesn't mind me saying so, for at least six months. And it doesn't totally have to do with us being new parents, zonk-tired, up at 4:00 a.m. It's partly due to the lack of spontaneity I feel when it comes to sex, now that I have one more thing (a fairly big thing, actually) to consider...besides time, place, baby feeding, who's gotta get up in the morning. I mean, I gotta think about going into the john, emptying, folding, and medi-taping my ostomy bag to my belly so it doesn't get in the way of, sorry, there's no other way to say it, Hon, thrusting.

golf and my cancer

Standing on the first tee at St. Andrews Old Course, 6:30 a.m., under leaden Scottish skies, one year after surgery, alone with my friend Renny on a course not yet open, here because he's pulled some strings, told some sad-true tale of an American friend who battled bowel cancer and came out of it alive, who's now waggling his Big Berthas and itching to play a round by the Firth of Forth (at the first available opportunity). As if the links gods are watching, kid you not a whit, there's a break in the clouds and the sun decides to join us on golf's shrine, if only for a moment.

the endorsement: the bag

Friend asks how everything's going—I can tell he means with the stoma, the ileostomy, the not-exactly-colostomy I had during surgery.... "Okay," I say. "I go to the gym, bike, hike, eat pretty much anything...." Turns out his mom's friend has a bag, got blocked up and she had to go to the hospital, twice, from peanuts. Twice??!! I'd give up the peanuts if I got blocked up once. Don't wanna know how the thing gets flushed.

choosing my religion

A Jewish family friend writes: "I don't know if you remember me, but I do you—When my mom had breast cancer, I didn't understand a lot of what she was going through. Reading your articles allowed me to feel it for the first time.... God chooses people he knows can handle it. He chose you...."

Thanks, God. Got my colon carved out in an eight-hour surgery, lost 45 pounds and nine months of my life in a freakish/mawkish/radiated/toxic-chemical/narcotics-infused blur of an assault, and as far as I know [sic], Osama's still doing fine, humpin' it round the Afghan/Pakistani border, with a leaky frickin' kidney. Still I pray.

nap time

Sometimes when Joshua sleeps in my arms, his warm head cradled in the crook of my elbow, I want to cry for the joy I feel.

Or maybe for the pain I didn't let myself feel when I thought I might die ahead of my time. And his.

stats all, folks

Two years post-op, two and a half since diagnosis, sitting on Doc Cohn's tissue-paper-covered leather table one more time. Learning, on April 22, 2003, that there are no lesions visible in my latest set of scans. He says I am healthy, then serves up a best-supporting statistic: "Eighty percent of the people who develop a recurrence [of colorectal cancer] get it in the first two years," he says. Which means just 20 percent develop it later.

Handshakes and hugs all around; pretty good odds, I figure. Until later that day, when I realize: Before I was first diagnosed, people like me, ex-colitis patients, had less than a 20 percent chance of developing colon cancer in the first dang place.... At the three-year mark [and at the big five-year CT in '06], my scans again appear medically "unremarkable." Which I—on the other hand, a few years after dealing with an elusive, shadowy death rattle—find rather remarkable.

Quick call to family, with Paula at my side; then dial best pal Geoff in L. A.

"I don't have can-cerrrrr, I don't have can-cerrrrr," I sort of white-man-rap at him. "I don't have can-cerrrrrrr!" Pause. Then he answers: "This month."

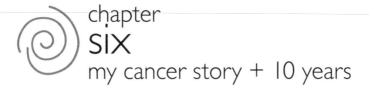

chapter
SIX
my cancer story + 10 years

stats all, folks

Ten years post-op, 10-and-a-half since diagnosis: Sitting on Denver Dr. Allen Cohn's tissue paper-covered leather exam table one more time. Learning, in October, 2011, that there are no lesions visible in my latest set of CT scans. Old NED, happy to say. *N.E.D.* as the medicos like to say. No Evidence of Disease, as we patients like very much—are you frickin' kidding me how very much—to hear. Doc says I am healthy, then goes on to say, I don't need to have any more annual CT scans to follow my decade-ago colorectal cancer diagnosis. "If we find something now, it's considered a new cancer," he says. Which brings me instant, heartfelt relief. But, honestly, this also makes me wonder, anew: "What the hell do you expect to find...'*now*'"?

my jewelry that's not

Guess it's been more than a year, now, that I've kept a simple yellow wristband on, the one that says LIVESTRONG, the one and I used to just wear every now and then. I don't wear it to protest anything cancer-specific. Don't wear it to tout any biological or medical miracle pride. Don't wear it, either, to support any single celebrity cyclist. (Disclosure: I have done some work for the LIVESTRONG Foundation, the one that used to go by the name: The Lance Armstrong Foundation. See Chapter Nine.) Don't even pretend to wear it to jumpstart (the rest of) my life. No, I wear the wristband 24/7 because I've found, after enduring chemotherapy, radiation, surgery, then more chemo, that the band connects me instantly to a community that means more to me personally than Facebook, LinkedIn, or Google+. Setting my own cancer case details temporarily aside (they're trumpeted all through Chapter 2), it's my faux-jewelry, plasti-rubberized accessory that gains me entry, time and again, and again, into the Survivors' Social Network. All it asks for, in return, is a little bit of real estate 'round my wrist. And some shampoo once in a while in the shower. Deal.

my good cancer year that's not

While I was diagnosed in December, then again in January for real, my last treatment wasn't completed until mid-September. So, technically speaking, My Good Cancer Year was more like nine months. But it took me at least another three months to get my taste buds back (chemo can screw with your tongue and all). And it took me a lot longer than three more months to get my confidence—if you could call it that—back. As for my physical fitness and sexual function, you ask? Well even if you hadn't, I'm being more honest than coy when I say: I'm still working on those. The good news is, the function is there. On both counts. (Again, pls. see Chapter 2.) The not-so-fantabulous news? I'm still working on those.

tumor in a bottle

Not sure i want to say "yes" to this idea, but how can I say *No*? I mean: How can I say no to a doctor who helped save my life? Not long ago I attended a Webinar (remotely, that is, via laptop +

headphones), at which Alan Venook, M.D., my medical oncologist at the University of California-San Francisco cancer center, was speaking. In fact he was speaking about my disease—colorectal cancer—and all the new treatments that are available today. I thought back: When I was diagnosed, there weren't half or even one-third the number of treatments for my particular type of cancer that now are possibilities. There basically were two drugs: 5-FU and Leucovorin. Times have changed, hope springs anew.* Yet despite huge gains in genomics and proteomics knowledge— the molecular biology of how cancers develop—1.6 million people are still diagnosed annually in the U.S. Yep, 1,600,000. Plus.

So yes, I sent an e-mail to my ex-doc, checking in and letting him know I'd seen his presentation. And he e-mailed back, almost instantly. He remembered me, for sure. We got to talking; and at one point he suggested it would be interesting to take a new look at my old tumor (housed in newfangled formaldehyde, I'm guessing, in some climate-controlled pathology labs), to see if and how I might have been treated differently today versus early in the 2000s. How could I say no? I could not. Although I'm not exactly looking forward to seeing my tumor tissue floating in a bottle, or swabbed onto a frozen slide, on my next trip to that hospital-o'-mine. No matter the why nor how.

....

* As of this writing, in 2013, the following drugs had been approved for use in treating colorectal cancer in the U.S.:

Bevacizumab (Avastin®); Capecitabine (Xeloda®); Cetuximab (Erbitux®); Fluorouracil, 5-FU (Adrucil); Irinotecan (Camptosar®); Irinotecan HCl Injection (Camptosar®); Leucovorin (Leucovorin); Levamisole (Ergamisol); Oxaliplatin (Eloxatin®); Panitumumab (Vectibix®); Stivarga Tablets (Regorafenib®); Ziv-Aflibercept Injection (Zaltrap®).

the right time for family time?

In a patient's or survivor's cancer world, timing isn't everything. But it's often way more important than you may realize—at the time. In my case, in our case, immediately after my diagnosis, a question came up whether we should go ahead with a scheduled interview with a social worker about future adoption plans—that now was set to happen 24 hours after my being diagnosed. Should we proceed with this...as planned? What we faced straight-damn-away was: Does it make sense now to talk about a future baby for this family when there may not be a future daddy? There were two ways to go that day, in regard to the appointment. Do we reschedule it, maybe for never? Or do we proceed with making plans for our family, cancer-or-no-cancer? Which I now realize, years later, is another way of saying:

Do we submit to cancer and all of its demands, 100 percent? Or do we keep control of a certain, important proportion of our lives, no matter the unsettled, scary, cancerous state of biology inside my skin and bones? Do we operate from here on...from a sense of fear? Or with a sense of optimism, tinged with both reality and fear?

We chose optimism. We met with the social worker. Our eldest son, Josh, is now one of the happiest, brightest, beloved 5th-grade boys that I know. (His younger brother, Jesse, would on most days agree with that assessment.) We went with Family before fear.

cry me a river

I'm not the kind of guy who cries a lot. At funerals, yes. At sad movies, okay, on occasion. Like three or four times a year. And, yes, after getting a diagnosis of cancer, I cried. Not immediately, not during the initial phone call from my doctor who performed the colonoscopy that found the cancer: Maybe that's because I couldn't take it all in at first. I didn't cry at first because I was in a sort-of-state-of-shock.

What I mean is: I'd had a screening, preventive colonoscopy a couple of years earlier, at age 40, due to family history (colon disease and cancer) and risk factors (ulcerative colitis), and apparently my goofball gastroenterologist at the time missed signs of evident cancer. This is what my more trusted, more pedigreed cancer surgeon told me later—that the cancer was at least five, maybe 8-to-10, years old. And that whoever had performed the earlier colonoscopy had missed the cancer that was present. Not "possibly" present. The earlier, GI doctor missed it. That's why I was so surprised about my initial diagnosis. That's why I think, looking back, that I didn't cry. Until later. Until my wife, Paula, came home and we talked together, alone in an otherwise empty house, about the cancer news I'd just received. I had cancer; and she, a 38-year-old movie producer who worked in the world of make believe, maybe wasn't fully prepared for this shock-reality medical news of the day. About her husband. The guy who now was crying, silently weeping-and-heave-breathing, in hopes that she wouldn't hear his muffled crying, amid her own louder, choke-breath sobs.

So, yes, absolutely. I cried that day. And I cried more than a few times over the next few months during some of the hardest, harshest parts of my treatment. From searing moments of pain, through the Why-Me must-get-throughs.

Nowadays, I try to suck it up and not cry when I get news of friends who get cancer diagnoses, now that I'm firmly middle aged. And need to be there for them. If I'm not the expert; at least I'm the shoulder to download upon. After prostate scares or diagnoses, I freely talk penises and erections with guy friends worried about their sexual and urinary futures. With gal friends, I talk about BrCA genes and HER-2 subtype diagnoses; and I find myself the recipient at times of late-night e-mails that detail the after-effects of breast surgery, lymph node adhesions, and lymphedema that follows.

Maybe I didn't sign up for this, but by publishing journal-blog entries in an *Esquire* six-part series during My Cancer Year, maybe I auditioned for the role by default. I went public. I took my intestines and colon and rectum—and my marriage and more—by extension, out of the radiation and chemo rooms and into the blogosphere. And beyond. So that's in part why people feel comfortable sharing their groan-and-groin stories with me. And that's partly why, oftentimes, I find myself *not* crying when I want to.

earth-shattering alert

It came without warning. Getting down on all fours one sunny San Francisco morning, for once not because of being nauseated, nor due to cancer pain that rendered me instantly horizontal. Not this a.m. It's a crack in the earth's crust sending a different sort of message, rendering me woozy, cautious, fawn-like, though low on the Richter scale.

Turns out I'm halfway through treatment by now, a transplanted Midwestern guy who grew up preparing for tornadoes not earthquakes. Who now finds my sick self swaying—slightly—in a century-old building, wondering how bad the quake needs to be before we gotta evacuate. Then it *stops*-quick. No reverb. And I realize how relatively unfrightened I was during my first earthquake. Turns out my diagnosis of Stage 3 cancer cells rocked my world more. "Is it over?" I wonder. "Is it done now, puh-leez," I think but don't say, "so I can get back to just being a cancer survivor?"

my genes, my *proteomes*, my family colons

As a blustery, Iraq War-era, U.S. Defense Secretary once said, "You go to war with the army you have, not the army you...wish to have at a later time." Roger that. Large-intestinally speaking, my maternal grandmother had colon cancer when she died in her 40s. My mother had ulcerative colitis and her colon surgically removed at age 75. And so I inherited, at least in part, a colon that was destined for trouble, big trouble, once I got a diagnosed with colitis in my 20s. My digestive disease war was on. They said I'd have to watch "this thing" all through my 30s and into my 40s. Which I did, but still got awarded with colon cancer at 43.

Looking back, looking ahead, it's nice to know that there's a company (SomaLogic) based in the town in which I live (Boulder, Colo.), where they are studying all the micro-factors that lead to cancer—in order to improve patients' odds in their future wars with cancer. Scientists here are searching far beyond the genome to the "proteome" (including tiny proteins and lifestyle factors by the *millions* that also influence who gets cancer and who doesn't). In my survivor's mind, it's better to have SomaLogic and it's ilk in town, than it is having another CorePower Yoga or Starbucks on the corner.

no red bull, either

Can't tell you exactly when it started, maybe four weeks after diagnosis. Maybe six: *No. Morning. Coffee.* After 20 years, more or less, of my drinking it daily. Timing wise, might have been after the radiation effects and nausea totally kicked in. But uh-*uh*. No more. No doctor's orders, either. Just couldn't deal. Also may have had something to do with the fact that I had moved out of my house, 1,250 miles west, to get some world class cancer treatment in San Francisco...and that I'd left my trusty Braun coffeemaker back at home. Or it might have been that my taste buds got fried-numbed-dulled from chemo; so what's the use of drinking fair-trade, praise-the-holy-farmer, organic coffee beans anyway, when you can't frickin' taste 'em? And if you do try—you might get sick anyway.

And so: No java, no a.m. jumpstarts for the better part of six-to-nine months. No Red Bull, either, now that I look back. No need for caffeine spark energy at this time. What I needed was: honest-a-goodness energy from oxygen carried by healthy red blood cells that I no longer had, during the fight of my life. Beyond EPO, the so-called red blood cell wonder drug, it would take time for some new daily addictions of mine, stronger meds, courtesy of the opiate Rx family, soon to take hold.... Little did I know at the time.

a friend kind of, sort of, wants to know, right?

It's a question that could have been answered either way.

Not long ago, a breast cancer survivor friend asked me: "It's all a numbers game, right?"

I didn't answer right away. Didn't know if she really even *wanted* me to answer. Every cancer is so damn different. Then I wondered if what she later wrote to me didn't answer her own question after all. In whip-smart poetic fashion, even:

"And in the end
you just have to do
what you do
with the info you have
and move on...."

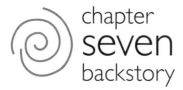

chapter
seven
backstory

cancerstory

A year or so after my journal-like takes about my cancer found their ways into magazineland, an ex-girlfriend of mine got hold of me from the East Coast. She did so a couple of decades after we had gone out, to tell me that she, too, had been diagnosed with cancer. Hers was breast cancer, seemingly under control now. And she wanted to tell me how she related to so much of what I seemed to be trying to say, even if my anger wasn't always out front or evident. She also said, or maybe I did: how weird it was that we now shared something else, apart and sort of together, as middle-aged ex-New Yorkers.

Weeks and months went by as we both adjusted to our newfound survivorship. She was divorced, I was married. She had to wend her way through treatment on her own. I did not. She decided to join a cancer advocacy group for support and to fight the fight in larger ways. I sat back, and didn't. At least at first. But I did later decide to approach *The New York Times* to ask whether they might want to publish a story of mine, about an unlikely modern relationship. They said yes. And so a "Modern Love" column about cancer, a guy, and a girl, made its way into the public eye on August 12, 2007:

as survivors, we were closer than lovers

Less than a minute after I arrived alone, via Amtrak from Manhattan, I knew this wasn't going to be easy. My ex-girlfriend, who was being as gracious as she could be after enduring a couple of years of cancer and four (partly successful) combinations of chemotherapy, was lighting a candle.

Or trying to. And it became clear in an instant: Her fingers wouldn't work. The matches kept bending, mushing, with each strike, before any whiff of sulfur. A side effect of her newfangled chemo regimen: neutropenia, neuropathy (or something similarly cruel-sounding) that deadens the nerves of patients' fingertips.

The candle was to be a nice touch, her warm way of welcoming me into her home, a loft in an artsy Philadelphia neighborhood where she went to live, and create, and create a new life for herself after her marriage, after the diagnosis, long after our short relationship.

But here we were together again, decades after our first hookup, because (we both knew but didn't say) there was a small chance this could be our last face-to-face meeting, our last hugs and goodbye. Especially if her next courses of breast cancer treatments didn't do what her A-list oncologist and the rest of us all hoped.

Cancer survivorship was the other reason we were together again. She got her diagnosis at 43, the same age that I received a diagnosis of colon cancer. She had volunteered with the Young Survival Coalition, and a year later spied my *Esquire* article about my ordeal.

After a Web search or three, she found me. Now we were writing, talking, sharing bits of our lives again, glad that both of us were able to talk about our midlives (which we realized could very well have been our late lives).

We were exes-in-remission, reminiscing, sharing stories of white blood cell loss, hair loss, weight loss and adventures in vomiting. A far cry from what we once had been: young, hungry, reckless-in-our-20s New York creative types, carving out a place for ourselves in the city of too many roommates and too much competition with those chasing all-too-similar dreams.

not enough visible love?

Dream over, she suddenly relapsed the year before last. And went to inform human resources at her creative job. And went on disability. Pain took command, along with unruly lesions that surfaced in her liver. Soon we both knew she was in for a long, wicked ride to, we hoped, remission 2.0. Time once again to board the slow chemo train, but this time with the newfound dread of less-forgiving odds—mixed like a medi-cocktail, with resolution, anger, hope. And not enough visible love, as even those closest to you at times pull away. Emotionally, physically.

It's uncomfortable at this point to say that I found a few of her notes flirtatious over the course of the last year; over the course of our chat-room-like e-mail messages minus the chat room. We were one-on-one. But especially as a guy in a good, solid marriage, I have no reason to lie: Once you sleep with someone, it's hard to ever get together with them again, no matter how much later, without thinking of the physical closeness that was, or wasn't quite, or might have been.

That's got to be the "love" in "making love" talking, even after so long, or else my thoughts of those long-ago nights spent together, so out of place in the here and now, wouldn't be troubling me today, amid all this sickness and sadness. I mean, should it take tumor metastases to allow us to fully feel such things and admit to them?

Back in her home, we took solace in the fact that we had made our own sort of mini support group, founded in part upon late-night e-mail notes and a call or two that consciously evaded mention of our long-ago love affair. There was a welcome lightness to our new friendship, a safe space.

When she pulls out the photo album, I ask, "Were we really that young?" ("Were we really that happy?" I think but don't say.) After a while she opens up and tells me a bit about her ex-boyfriend: the one who left soon after her diagnosis, telling her he didn't think he was the "caregiver type," though she claims her disease didn't cause their split.

My face crumples, incredulous, in protest. "Hey, at least I found out early on he wasn't The One," she says, in a more forgiving tone than I'd ever be able to muster. Later she adds, "It's sad that cancer had to be the catalyst." But now she's talking about how it brought the two of us together again.

Maybe so. But we also know that without our cancer, we probably never would have been together again. And certainly not like this: amid all the trappings of what might seem to outsiders like a romantic reunion, yet one that is socially permissible, even encouraged, given the circumstances.

shred the polite filters!

These days, I find that survivor friendships like ours make you confront, early and often, the heavy and the light, and in so doing you find you are granted a curious kind of freedom. You shred the polite filters. You get a pass to cut to the chase. Because time together means more now.

After all, we became instantly closer in our mid-40s than we ever were in our early 20s, when she was an up-and-coming design student in art school, and I was a journalist sending all manner of suck-up notes to contacts at *Newsweek*, *BusinessWeek*, *Rolling Stone*, while trying to type my way out of trade journalism.

One bright fall day more than 20 years ago, she and I hopped a New York bus to the New Jersey Palisades. Over the George Washington Bridge we rolled, without having packed a lunch, or lugging even a single plastic water bottle (urbanites didn't yet hydrate like that). We went to walk some paths, take some pictures (in arty black-and-white), crunch some leaves under our desert boots. We made out a little, in PG-13 fashion, shrouded by a stand of stubborn oaks that hadn't shed their leaves on schedule.

Now, on another brisk fall day, two major diagnoses later, sharing herbal tea in her urban loft space, we dish about magazines and photographers she knows; more about new times than old; about how parts of our bodies didn't (or don't) work so well when we were (or are) fighting our cancers. We don't say anything at all about how we broke up, or much about our current love lives, or family lives, either. I feel "survivor's guilt" hanging heavy in the room, thinking it's unfair that I'm cancer free, five years after my nasty Stage 3, and she's suffering through the muck of her now-Stage 4, after reaching remission three years ago.

No guarantees, we know but don't say, for either of us. Let's do today. Out of my backpack I share four magazines: *Interview*, *Vogue*, *Entertainment Weekly*, *Vanity Fair*. These, I had hoped, would appeal to the former art student who had lived in the Village near N.Y.U. with two other post-punk roommates when the Clash were the Coldplay of their time. She thanks me for bringing these pieces of the outside world in. Though now I wonder: If her fingers didn't work so well with soft matches, will they be able to easily flip 1,000 flimsy pages of advertising and articles? Will her eyes be able to handle the small type?

She's wearing glasses now, low on the bridge of her nose. She's wearing a wig, too, I see, although she doesn't mention it. She's also, through all this unfairness, looking somehow sexy to me, again. And this uninvited thought makes me feel old, confused, sad. But why shouldn't she? Are Stage 4 survivors not supposed to care how they look? What I know is: I hugged her so gently when I came through the doorway. Her body felt frail, unsteady, birdlike.

In the fading afternoon light we talk for some time about her travels, her passion for Italy, Elsa Schiaparelli, and other things artful.

Including some Euro-style photo shoots she had produced in the past few years while in her post-cancer prime. After we order takeout Italian supper ("I don't drive these days," she says), we make our way into her bedroom, carrying brown paper sacks and fragile wine goblets.

Only then do I remember: When you have cancer and your body's racked from chemo (and serious opioids for pain), entertaining is hard. Even when it's an old boyfriend who believes he's low maintenance, who's been through this himself, who's supposed to know you don't stay more than two or three hours on these kinds of visits. You just don't. Because it's hard on stage-whatever patients—it upsets their (our) routines in the middle of such long low-light days.

As we move to, and onto, her bed, she one-handedly swings a stylish tray table over for us to share. I take note: This is a woman who's been taking many of her meals on this same Scandinavian tray table.

"Welcome to my Capri bed," she says, smoothing the tufted comforter. What she means is: She took the money she had been saving for a (canceled) trip to Capri and bought this remote control bed instead.

I settle in, best I can, in the cold and dark next to her. Then I immediately bounce back up to forage for napkins, trying to be useful. With our fingers we eat pizzetta; with our eyes we blankly watch CNN. Then we talk a little about, God help us, Joe Biden's politics. And a comfortable silence envelops us, despite the nonstop cable chatter. It's a reconnection, a spark, however slight.

I take a swirl-sip of the fragrant French wine that my ex-girlfriend has just poured for me. Didn't notice: was it from a "good year"? No real reason to ask. Pretty much every year seems a good year about now. My back hurts a little as we sit scrunched side by side, moving our forks around. Outside, windblown leaves dance in the dark. Then I take another sip of, I don't know, Bordeaux. I can't taste it. I can't taste anything.

©*The New York Times*, reprinted by permission

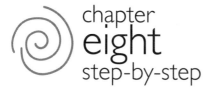

chapter
eight
step-by-step

Almost goes without saying: There's more than one way to fight cancer, no matter your prognosis. Question is: Which path, or paths, will you take? A team or support group approach? Or a more stand-it-alone? With or without a clinical trial? At the 10-year-plus mark of my survivorship, I decided to ditch the go-it-alone and reach out a little bit to others. Decided to get just a bit more serious about what it means to be a cancer survivor. So yes, I had the yellow wristband on, when I trained to enter the annual Bolder Boulder 10-kilometer run in 2011. Question also was: Could I get my ass back into something like 10-minutes-a-mile shape? The *Runner's World* editors were kind enough to let me train and track my journey as a survivor in some of their pages. The story ran in July, 2011.

still running
What cancer abruptly took away,
a race in the Rocky Mountains gives back, slowly but surely

When I crawled out of the foxhole of advanced, Stage 3 colon cancer in early 2001, I was 43 years old and had lost 35 pounds since the first drop of a 24/7 chemo combo first began pumping through my system. Bones wedged through depleted muscles and wasted skin. My "package" had become blackened by radiation's friendly fire upon the skin near my groin. My body, the one I had known so well for so many years, now felt like it belonged to an alien.

And to think that three months before my diagnosis I could still knock out a five-mile training loop near my Colorado home, at an altitude of some 6,000 feet, at a workmanlike but agreeable pace of 10 minutes per mile. Sure, some days it seemed I was getting winded sooner, that the workout felt more like a mile-high slugfest than the usual midday breeze.

no runner's high?

But I chalked that up to the sluggishness I'd been feeling of late, a sluggishness that my doctor thought was anemia. Nothing that a few iron pills couldn't cure, right?

I soon learned that there is no runner's high when you're fighting for your life. In my case, beyond my main tumor, there was, as the doctors cryptically reported, "lymph node involvement." In treatment early on, five or six times each day, I suffered self-rated nine out of 10 tumor pain that corkscrewed its way from the deepest realms of my bowels up my spinal cord and into my brain. It laid me horizontal—onto the nearest couch, bed, or bench (if I'd happened to escape out in public).

It was only after being eight weeks removed from surgery, and after chemo and radiation, that I decided to get vertical one June morning and gauge my post-cancer fitness. I thought I might be able to jog the friendly, 1.5-mile trail that rings Wonderland Lake in North Boulder. During my first 10 steps, though, I realized that even jog-walking a quarter-mile was out of the question. With pinkened scar tissue from my chest to my pubic bone (still more raw than I'd expected after two months), each step on the packed dirt and cinders sent shocks up my torso. So I stopped running, and did, maybe, two-tenths of a mile in a radiated survivor's shuffle. Then back home to lie down. Stat. Defeated.

Cancer can do that to you; it can make you forget that at one point, not so long ago, you ran a 10-K at altitude in 53:50.

I needed a plan. A long-term recovery plan. After all, I wanted badly to be moving again. I wanted to run from cancer, as fast as I could, as fast as my scar tissue and internal adhesions would let me. Posting mileage and 10-minute miles would mean I'm a human again, and not a full-time, sorry-assed cancer patient. A runner instead of a survivor. I considered chasing new, post-cancer PRs as a way to regain parts of my self that the disease stole from me. But before I could go there, I had an even bigger number to worry about.

Near the end of my treatment, I said to my oncologist, "Doc, what are my, um, chances?" I didn't use the word "survival," but he knew full well what I meant.

"Hard to say," the doctor replied rather benignly. "You're younger and stronger than most patients with this disease." All things considered, he told my wife and me, "you have perhaps a 60 percent chance of being alive in five years."

That's it? I thought. *Maybe 60 percent?*

He tried to clarify the situation. If I made it through Year Two cancer-free, he said, my odds would get even better. That's because of all colon-cancer recurrences, 80 percent happen within the first two years following surgery.

If anything, I at least had some target to latch on to. A finish line, of sorts. And with it I gingerly returned to the gym to do light weights, the cross-trainer machine, some do-it-yourself yoga stretches.

Only my prescribed, every-three-month scans and exams reassured me—and let me stretch my goals. First, loop the damn 1.5-mile lake. Then aim for a friendly 5-K. Then, fingers crossed, chase something close to stamina. I would enter the Bolder Boulder 10-K, a race I used to do each year before all the drama. My chief hope was to finish sub-60 minutes, as I'd done pre-diagnosis. If I could do that, maybe I could convince myself that maybe I could outrun this disease.

Emotionally, during my early return to running, I weathered the opposite of runner's high. I often felt post-workout lows, and often all alone. I was hurting, still. I was slow. But I didn't want to blame it all on cancer. I didn't want to wave the Cancer Survivor's flag, either. I wanted to put cancer in my rearview. Nothing against the pink ribbons and all, but I wanted to hurt "normally," like a runner who absentmindedly forgets his glucosamine.

I returned to the Bolder Boulder in May 2004 with thousands of other runners who, like me, had made the race an annual rite. They had their own reasons for coming back each year, but I only worried about my own, and what I needed to finish and go home satisfied. By then I was "N.E.D.," as the good docs often say in CT scan reports: No Evidence of Disease. Nothing could get me down...except my finishing time that morning: 1:03:48.

Cancer can do that to you: age you prematurely—in a heavy-legs, stiff-hip way—and make you wonder, will I ever be myself again?

It would take several years, and a lot of mileage, before I felt a few glints of speed during intervals and some strength actually return in my quads. Then, after forever it seemed, in the 2007 Bolder Boulder, I finally finished under an hour, in 58:50. A year later, 58:36. A year later, whoops, a 64:32. But that was okay. That year I had garden-variety plantar fasciitis pain in my left foot. Yes, a real runner's ailment.

Looking back, it was that race, the Bolder Boulder, more than the positive CT scans, or blood-count reports, or encouraging doctor's words, that allowed me to turn the corner toward normal. A simple race that gave me the complex answer I sought.

So when I pinned on my entrant's bib for the race in spring 2010, I chose not to add a tag that had been offered when I picked up my number; the tag would identify me as a cancer survivor out on the course. I just wanted to blend in. And for more than half the race, that's what I did. I passed some runners, and got passed by others, and checked my splits, and just ran. But then, heading east and away from the Rocky Mountains, near the five-mile marker and water stop, I suddenly found myself shouting, inexplicably, toward the Gatorade volunteers: "I'm a CANCER SURVIVOR!" Then I yelled it again, punching my fist skyward and grabbing a cup of electrolytes: "A SURVIVOR!"

Cancer can do that to you.

I can't explain why those words came out of my mouth. They startled me, the guy who said them. I've never joined a support group along with my colorectal cancer "peeps." Nor have I received post-cancer therapy. Yet sometimes, it seems, you can only hold in what you've been holding in for so long. I'm a Survivor.

I know I told myself I was running to be normal again. But if one day you find yourself running solo and screaming hugely, in an event a full decade after you got a life-threatening diagnosis and ended up weeping on the kitchen floor with your wife who's just collapsed in your arms at the shock of it all, well, sometimes you've got to admit that cancer never really leaves your life all the way. Like 100 percent. Sometimes you find, 10 years after your life took a horrible wrong turn, that you may be cancer-free but you're still running from it. And always will be.

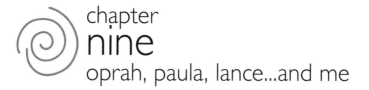

chapter
nine
oprah, paula, lance...and me

In July of 2010, Oprah Winfrey, via her *O* magazine (oprah.com/omagazine.html) decided to honor my wife and her colleagues by publishing a story about Paula's organization, There With Care (TWC), which is dedicated to helping children and families facing critical illness. By Oprah and Co. standards, Paula was a "hero" for the hundreds of families she and her staff and volunteers had served through their toughest of times, from providing transportation, meals, baby-sitting and home services help, to keeping families, cars and homes running despite taxing times in cancer hospitals, as this all had occurred on Paula's watch, ever since she founded TWC in 2005 as a Colorado-based nonprofit. (A Bay Area chapter opened in Northern California in 2012.)

Not surprisingly, the magazine mentioned Paula's other work, her work in Hollywood, because it's an odd combination of skills and services: helping families through cancer crises; and also helping movie makers through their own creative crises while beswamped by multi-million-dollar budget commitments and constraints.

I think of her mostly as my wife. But yes, Oprah, I will also remember all that she heroically did for me, all that's detailed back in Chapter 1, and all that she did for me that ended up on the cutting room floor, that didn't make it into these pages. Through it all, we became a rock-solid family that now will forever be bonded as well by *survivorship*. Which brings me to a different day...a different year, the year before There With Care served its first family. Turns out I was looking to make unlikely or unconventional connections, as well....

On October 4, 2004, I drove more than 40 miles to Denver to see six-time Tour de France champion (and cancer survivor) Lance Armstrong ride less than one mile on his bike. I went mostly to show support of his maiden, cross-country "Tour of Hope" charity ride, designed to improve the lives of countless cancer patients, survivors and their families. But truth be told, I also attended to find out what it feels like to "join" the fraternity of survivors in person, instead of merely in print. At work sometimes, at neighborhood barbecues; to many people I don't know that well, I'm "that guy who had colon cancer." At the Armstrong event, I'd be just another cancer dude, one among hundreds. Under leaden skies, unusual for Colorado that time of year, I climbed a short hill to get a better view, and watched the motorcycle police escort—all serious-like, in formation with swirling-flashing cop lights—part the milling crowd of about 2,000 people as they led Lance and his entourage to a podium behind the University of Colorado's Health Sciences Cancer Center. It felt pretty comfortable; I certainly wasn't alone.

After a couple quick warm-up jokes (including an unscripted dig at our leaders for spending $200 billion on Iraq instead of on cancer research at home), Armstrong thanked the crowd, his doctors, his fellow riders and the millions who'd bought the dollar LIVESTRONG wristbrands his foundation has sold. He then thanked the Bristol-Myers Squibb company for making the chemotherapy drugs that helped save his life. Then he left, too soon it seemed. I wanted more; I wanted to feel the (then-powerful) Armstrong "aura." Even though, I realized, after starting his Tour in California the week prior, he was only as far as the Rockies... and he had to pedal his self to Washington, D.C., with other survivor-cyclists, by next week. So I understood. I picked up my free energy bars, anti-cancer brochures and bottle of spring water and took off.

"On a bicycle, you never know what's around the next bend," Armstrong has said, "when a view may open up, or [when] the Alps may shear off into the sea."

lance and me, then and now

Sometimes, sitting in front of a laptop or tablet, you also don't know what's coming around the next bend. For in 2009, I received an e-mail and a call from New York City, from a company called Spot On Media, asking if I would be interested in launching and editing a magazine about and for cancer survivors, on behalf of the LIVESTRONG/Lance Armstrong Foundation.

Before saying yes, I remember thinking: "There aren't many media jobs where having had cancer is a bonus credential." Soon enough, I signed on, met hundreds of memorable survivors, care providers, and sources, and helped steer survivorship medicine, at least a little, as a media advocate.

And soon enough thereafter, in fall, 2012, I was working, putting finishing touches on the 15th Anniversary Issue of LIVESTRONG's magazine, and wondering how Lance Armstrong's reputation would hold up through the latest steroid and other performance enhancing drug-use charges levied against him. Before long, my staff and I saw what was coming around the bend. And it wasn't good news for a great foundation. Armstrong was banned from cycling and triathlon competitions by anti-doping watchdog officials for allegedly using banned substances during his career.

A few months later, Lance appeared on the Oprah Winfrey Network (there she goes again!), to answer questions about what he did and did not do that was illegal, and why, en route to winning a recordsetting, seven consecutive Tour de France races from

1999-2005. All of which he won as a cancer survivor. Needless to say, Oprah didn't call Lance a hero that night (nor the next night, for part 2 of the interview). And that is understandable. It wasn't her job those nights.

And yet...in over 15 years of service, the foundation that Armstrong built has served hundreds of thousands of people who care about cancer patients and survivors. And without defending or apologizing for his actions, I cannot name another athlete who has done so much for so many, starting when he did before he was famous or even well-known. (Again, this is not a defense of his training misdeeds, but a mention of an often under-reported fact.) You can say Lance the cyclist cheated during his cycling career. He's admitted that.

You can also say Lance the cancer patient cheated death. But you cannot in good standing say he and his foundation haven't helped hundreds of thousands of patients, survivors, and their families since the foundation started in 1997. At last count, three films about Armstrong were said to be in the works following his ban from major sports.

Lance, and Oprah. And Paula and Oprah. And cancer. And, yes, Hollywood. How did we get here, again? All in these pages and screens?

going round the next bend

In fact I wrote this book to help survivors and their families navigate the territory "round the next bend"—whether that means four months till the next CT scan...or four years till cancer-free "cure." I also wrote this book because I believe every cancer patient can take a bit more control of his or her body, in a positive way. But don't take it from me: Listen to Dr. Barrie Cassileth, an expert in healing therapies at Memorial Sloan-Kettering Cancer Center, when she told me, in speaking of acupuncture: "We used to think the gains were due to a placebo effect. But that can't be said to be true for children and animal studies, and they have both shown positive effects." Pets, after all, simply have no way of "faking" feeling better. I wrote this book because the terrain of healing is changing as well, and most every survivor can use (at least parts of) a field guide of sorts.

As survivors and patients in the 2010s, we now know major advances have been made since 1995 in terms of curing and managing colorectal cancer. And while colon cancer may still lag behind breast and prostate cancer in the public consciousness and research dollars, it's gaining. And quickly. Where surgeons and doctors used to have just a few choices when it came to treating their patients for breast or colorectal cancer, some now bemoan there are too many choices! In some ways the science has outstripped the practice of medicine. The proof is that docs admit they often aren't sure which drug to use first. But as doctors and patients (and their families) have told me or shown me time and again in these pages, there is more than a little reason to be optimistic. As I've come to learn, as a former patient who once was starving just to hear that I was potentially curable, there is real reason to believe that in our lifetimes, cancer will lose and survivors will win.

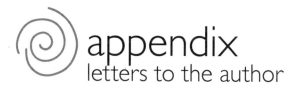

appendix
letters to the author

Date: Fri, 4 Jun 2004 07:50:15 EDT
From: <Scou@aol.com>
To: <curtpmail@aol.com>
Subject: another article

"Cancer Deaths Down in U.S., Report Finds"

WASHINGTON (June 3) — More Americans are surviving cancer for five years or more and cancer rates overall are steadily declining, according to the latest annual report on cancer in the United States issued on Thursday.

Talk About It

• Post Messages
• Top News Boards

[Author's note: Yes, Scou@aol.com. We will, Scou. We will Talk About It.]

From the time I learned I had advanced colorectal cancer, through nine months of treatment, through writing about what it felt like, through the 3-year mark of "all-clear" follow-up tests and scans, I received more emotional letters, e-mails and postcards, by far, than I did in 43 years of life prior to my life-threatening diagnosis. Writing, it turns out, can be more than therapeutic for many a cancer patient. It can be life-affirming. A handful of the most memorable, and of those perhaps most helpful to other survivors, appears below*.

from *Esquire* magazine's july, 2001, issue, letters-to-the-editor page:

"Fighting Cancer"

Our May issue…featured the first part of an ongoing series by Curtis Pesmen on his battle with colon cancer ("My Cancer Story: Part One").

I picked up *Esquire* several times this past week, and each time I put it down. Fear made me do it—the fear that the word cancer spreads. But finally Pesmen's words seduced me, and I found myself devouring his piece, wanting to understand every emotion and physical sensation he felt. Part of that was self-defense; part of it came from reading a piece that pierced the armor I carry to shield myself from the idea of disease. When I finished, I picked up the phone and called my doctor, whom I hadn't seen in a couple of years, and said, "I'm 35, and I want a full checkup." He said, "Wise move." I said a friend suggested it. If courage and bravery count for anything, Pesmen will kick cancer's ass.

—*Richard Abate, New York, NY*

*(Note: some names have been abbreviated or deleted, for privacy reasons.)

letter from a stranger, april, 2001:

Dear Mr. Pesmen,

It's Easter Sunday morning as I write.... Although I'm not a religious person, my faith in humankind is a bit restored as a result of your writing Part I in *Esquire*. Like your friend's daughter wished you, ... "I hope you fight off your cancer."

On an action-taking note, I'm 62 years of age and tomorrow I will call for a sigmoidoscopy exam. So thanks for being the impetus for my doing what is overdue. With sincere wishes for a full recovery and the very best for you and your wife.

—T.R.

letter from a friend, april, 2001, one week after stressful, successful, eight-hour surgery:

Dear Curt and Paula,

Well, I'm sure you have heard every bit of consolation, hope and now finally praise. Count me among the grateful. Thousands thanking God this day and just about every after for the good news that broke last week.

There are few people in the world who bring with them such calm and good will as Curt brings with him. I don't know if that is because we have sat next to each other at various functions and he lets me yammer on, that could be. But I have heard other people say the same thing about him and I am inclined to believe it is a genuine good disposition. Count me among the fortunate for knowing a wonderful person like Curt.

For two people to be in such an extreme position and display their love to each other in caring and patience, and for showing the immortal strength of love, count me among the believers.

Before you guys left [before the diagnosis], Paula and I were talking about her particular skill in the work place...and her ability to keep a cool head and manage multiple tethers, numbers, personalities and information. For Paula's being able to handle the circus of appointments, treatments and doctors without flinching or buckling, count me among the amazed.

While you may find this a bit much, I didn't know how else to let you both know how much you mean to me and just how happy I am that Curt is on the mend. I realize that there is more work ahead for you both, but know that we are still thinking about you, and will continue to root for speed on your road to recovery.

Love you both, and so very happy—
Booey

from an old colleague, young cancer survivor, and friend, may, 2001:

Dear Curt,

That's a hell of a way to have a two-part [sic] feature in *Esquire!*

Curt, I am so sorry to hear about your cancer. I read your pieces with my heart in my mouth and tears in my eyes. So much of what you said mirrored my own experience with breast cancer four years ago. And, although the whole thing completely sucks, I'm so grateful that you have a strong, loving partner with whom to go through it.

One thing you didn't mention was whether you had friends or support group pals who also had cancer and are our age. I felt with breast cancer that, because it's so politicized and so feminist-y, I fell into this ready made community of supportive women and it really helped me. Just to have someone to talk to, to vent with, someone who is not your spouse and doesn't have quite that emotional investment, someone who is going through it or has gone through it, someone who can hear your darkest fears without panicking.

And I wanted you to know that if you ever need to talk to someone about [being] a young person with cancer, my number is at the top of this page. That's it. I wish you the best of luck, the best of health, the best of love and all the strength you need.

Much love,
Peggy O., California

from a not-quite-friend of a friend, may, 2001:

Dear Curt,

You may not know me…but my father was diagnosed with a rare form of skin cancer when he was just approaching 45 and I was 17 at the time and I can remember that it was the 1st time I saw my father cry. Sometimes my Mom and Dad would just sit on the couch and start crying together. I could not really understand that at the time and it made me feel so awkward to see that and not know what to say or do. I remember the frustration in their voices…and it seems like everybody is polite to you but also scared to talk to you in fear that you may want to talk about "it," and that would just make us so uncomfortable.

Mmmhhh, let's think on that one… makes "us" uncomfortable?? Hell, there is nothing wrong with "us" now, is there? What about the person with the darn cancer, ever thought how uncomfortable they are—physically, emotionally and overall just uncomfortable knowing this damn cancer has invaded their body without their consent and often for a long time without them ever knowing?

Have we ever stopped to think how uncomfortable "YOU" must be? No, we tend to be selfish and think of us first and foremost and yes, then there is the thought of others...and how sorry we may feel about them and how tragic that someone we know may be sick, but followed right away by the afterthought, "Thank God it is not me!" How selfish can we get? It wasn't until a couple years ago that I understood that concept of thinking when I witnessed a good friend of mine die of AIDS. Not a pretty sight....

Curt—you and Paula are in my deepest prayer tonight and every night and I sure hope that I will have the pleasure of getting to meet both of you one day.

Best wishes,
S.E., North Carolina

from a friend of a friend, who lives in st. louis:

Dear Curt,

When I had cancer five years ago, I was sure I'd be dead by now. I spent a lot of hours crying about my children being raised without me, etc., and giving my sister and my husband lots of instructions. I even listed the single friends who would make acceptable stepmothers. Any time anyone told me I looked good—a complete lie as my skin was green during chemo, and my hair is one of my best features—I would say, "Open Casket."

Ignore everyone's advice, but here's some anyway: Avoid all books that tell you to have a positive attitude. Wallow—you've more than earned it. Wishing you all the best. If I had crystals, I'd use them—that is, after someone explained to me what the hell they're supposed to do.

Part of my nightmare was that my kids were 8 and 5, and one of my parents died when I was 8, but if we're going to throw around cancer psycho-babble, my guess is that losing a body part, like a breast, is a pretty tangible daily reminder. Even to someone who has had her plastic surgery redone numerous times.

Not that I'm trying to one-up you or anything. Here's an anecdote to cheer you up: The goofball husband of an old friend of mine had testicular cancer the same time I had breast cancer. Whenever he felt especially freaked out, he would call me to "commiserate," but really to work into the conversation that his cancer had a 98 percent cure rate, unlike mine. Not that I'm the sort of person to hold a grudge.

Best, Jill F.

from *Esquire*'s september, 2001, issue, letters page, "the continuing battle":

July also brought the third installment in Curtis Pesmen's ongoing account of his fight with colorectal cancer ("My Cancer Story").

I am 40. I have brain cancer. I was diagnosed in April and was operated on five days later, and have seven radiation treatments to go. Hats off to Pesmen for sharing his experience with us all. It isn't easy to read, but cancer isn't easy to have. I've learned a lot, but mostly that fatigue and nausea are the two most misrepresented words in the English language. Good stuff, but damn, I'm mad. Seven months ago, I ran a marathon. And I guess, just like Pesmen, I don't want to die.

—T.T., Richmond, Va.

from a writer friend in new york, with whom I had some tough words in the spring of 2001:

Dear Curt,

Thanks a million for calling last night…. You asked me why I wanted to reach out to you when I haven't done so with others in the past. I think the simple answer is: It's about you. With other people I've often been afraid that my expressions of sympathy would sound like I was just projecting my own fears, like the way people who cry at weddings are overwhelmed by their own romantic ideals, not the reality of someone else's life. I've been afraid there was something phony about forging a close relationship with someone only after they contracted a serious disease. Even in your case I couldn't help wondering if you thought your writer friends might try to use you in a Mitch Albom-esque way.

The difference here is that I know you. We may be closer to other people than we are to each other, but I feel for sure that over the years we've moved past the friends-of-friends status to being just friends, and I certainly know you well enough to have genuine feelings for you as a person…. And it's not just a personal loss for me; I know too how many people you've touched and what the loss of you would mean to them.

So now back to our mutual insensitivities: what have we learned from all this? How about: I promise not to say any more obnoxious things if you promise not to have any more cancer.

Still your friend,
Ben

an e-mail from a friend in new york, upon learning of the death of a young friend of mine, july, 2004:

Curt,

You know, I'm beginning to believe that it's the norm and not heroic for people to keep fighting and stay optimistic when they are really ill (not that I can tell YOU how people act when they are ill...). But truly, I've yet to run in to anyone who has a dire illness who DOESN'T rally to live and fight on. Part of this is because we don't see them when they are curled up in a ball in the corner of the room petrified of what's to come.

But I do find this so inspiring.... Imagine: it's not "normal" for a person who is dying to become morbid; it is "normal" for the human spirit to fight back and stay "up" for everyone around them. Remember the last thing you wanted was for people to think of you as "Cancer Boy," so the only way to ensure that is to act like you are NOT sick.... Makes sense, no?

Are you okay?
—H.

from an old pal, ex-girlfriend, and breast cancer survivor, who read an article of mine and reached out my way, spring 2007:

Curt—

I always felt badly about the fact that you were the unfortunate recipient of so much of my own unfiltered deeply depressing stuff I couldn't talk to my other "real-world" friends about...that they didn't want to hear and/or didn't understand. [You know,] its sadly too rare that we ever get to know what "exes" really thought about anything.

xo, s.

from my father, then 72, after an early-morning airport departure following his four-day visit during my chemo:

Dearest Children,

You two have given me such optimism-courage-support I feel like I'm the one who is winning the battle!

I love you both so much—
Dad

from *Esquire* magazine's october, 2001, issue, letters page, "on the road to recovery":

In August, Pesmen continued with the fourth part of his series on his fight against colon cancer.

I have been an *Esquire* subscriber for more than 30 years. I keep renewing because I feel that *Esquire* deals intelligently with issues affecting men. My faith has been reinforced by your publication of Curtis Pesmen's "My Cancer Story." I was diagnosed with colon cancer more than seven years ago. I have read all of Pesmen's articles and think that he has been able to convey the emotions that I felt during my diagnosis and treatment. His article, however, is just the beginning of the fight, as cancer is never cured but only goes into remission.

For the rest of his life, every little ache, fever or other change in his body will bring concerns that the monster has returned. If it does, as has mine has, a new set of feelings will come. I realize that I will eventually die of cancer and it is important to make every day enjoyable. It appears that Pesmen has the most important tool needed to cope with his illness and prolong his life—a loving, caring, and supportive wife.

—*T.B., Metairie, La.*

Curtis Pesmen, a Colorado-based writer and content producer, is author of six books of non-fiction, including *How a Man Ages*, *What She Wants*, and *Your First Year of Marriage*. He has written or edited for *Esquire*, *Outside*, CNNMoney.com, *SELF*, *SPORT*, *The New York Times* and *CURE*. He also has served as founding editor of *LIVESTRONG Quarterly*, co-founder of WidowsList.com, and often speaks and writes on patient advocacy issues. He lives with his wife and family in Boulder, Colorado.